Forget the Viagra ...

Pass Me a Carrot!

Nothing Personal!
Best wishes and hugs
Sally x

by

Sally Cronin

Forget the Viagra ... Pass me a Carrot!
Sally Georgina Cronin
E-mail:- sallygcronin@gmail.com
Skype:- Moyhill2

Website:- http://www.moyhill.com/FTV
http://www.amazon.co.uk/-/e/B003B7O0T6
Daily health blog:-
http://ftvpmac.wordpress.com

Moyhill Publishing

Published by Moyhill Publishing.

ISBN 978-1-905597-42-0

A CIP catalogue record for this book is available from the British Library.

Printed in UK.

Designed & typeset by *Moyhill* Publishing.

The papers used in this book were produced in an environmentally friendly way from sustainable forests.

Moyhill Publishing,
Suite 471, 6 Slington House,
Rankine Rd., Basingstoke, RG24 8PH, UK

Contents

Contents ...

Contents ...

Contents . . .

Health Warning

NHS website on Cardiovascular disease

- Cardiovascular disease is the leading cause of death both in the UK and worldwide.
- In the UK over 1.6 million men and women are affected by Chronic Heart Disease.
- It is responsible for more than 88,000 deaths in the UK each Year, or 224 people each day, which is one person dead every 6 minutes.
- Most deaths from heart disease are caused by heart attacks – around 124,000 yearly.
- There are also 152,000 strokes each year in the UK resulting in 43,000 deaths.

Poor diet, lack of exercise and smoking
are the root causes of these deaths.

- Ignorance is not a defence
- Heart disease is a silent killer
- It is *your* responsibility to give your body a fighting chance by embracing a healthier lifestyle.

If you have not recently been examined by a doctor and are considering buying any sexual medication over the Internet – *think again* and go and get checked out first.

Your body is your greatest asset,
if you abuse it you lose it.

This book is not just about your sex life.
It is about your life.

How to Use This Health Manual

I have often used the car analogy when talking about the body and nutrition.

Imagine that you have a very high end, expensive car with all the bells and whistles and the first thing that any car enthusiast is going to do is pop the bonnet lid and take a look at the magnificent performance engine.

Your body is far more sophisticated than any muscle car and is a miracle of intricate systems and chemical reactions all designed to perform to a very high spec.

Like any piece of machinery it requires a very specific mix of nutrients and oils to fire on all cylinders.

You may very well know the inside of your car's engine intimately, but how well do you know your own body and how it functions? A body, which unlike a car that might last you ten years, has to remain fit and active for perhaps 90 years.

The first part of the book is the workshop manual and hopefully will give you an insight into the incredible job your organs and systems are undertaking every second, minute, hour of every day of your life.

The second part tells you about the components of the fuel necessary to drive this amazing engine.

The third part tells you the source of the nutrients in foods and fluids and shows you how to get the right mix specific to your particular engine and workouts for your engine.

Understanding how your body works and what you need to give it to be healthy and vital for as many years as possible, will also help prevent most of the common health issues associated with sexual decline.

I cannot promise you a terrific sex life but I hopefully will show you something that give you a sense of empowerment and control over your own health and wellbeing.

Part One

Introduction

I apologise in advance if you have picked up this book under the mistaken impression that I am going to be talking about sexual aids.

But, having got your attention, perhaps you would read the next couple of pages so that you can grasp the intent behind the title. I am afraid I am not offering a quick fix or an instant erection but rather a slightly longer term approach to enhancing and maintaining a healthy sex life into your 80's and 90's.

In fact this book is not just about getting your sex life on track but your health in general as this is one of the most likely cause of any problems now or in your future with sexual performance.

There seems to be some confusion as to who is responsible for the level of obesity and ill health we are currently suffering from and which is only going to get worse in generations to come. In fact they estimate that 75% of serious illnesses are lifestyle related.

The good news is that it is you the individual who is responsible and if you want to have a long and active sex life then you need to review your current lifestyle and make some decisions about your future.

I chose the title of my book as it seems that our sex lives seem to be the main focus and thrust of spammers these days, if you will pardon the pun.

Anyone who uses a computer and has access to the Internet will no doubt be bombarded with offers to supply Viagra or similar sexual performance enhancers at vastly deflated prices from various parts of the world.

Because my name is on the web in relation to health and nutrition I seem to get a double dose of this shotgun approach to selling drugs and it was while I was binning the 20th spam mail on the subject of the day that it occurred to me that perhaps a different message was in fact being sent to me.

I have been a practising nutritional therapist for over fifteen years and ran a dietary advisory clinic in Ireland. Both in Spain for the last five years and now back in the UK, I have provided healthy living programming for radio and also written articles and columns for magazines and other publications. I am a Life and Nutritional coach and whereas in the past most of my clients would have consulted me for weight issues, I now find myself designing eating and exercise programmes for couples who are facing fertility problems, patients preparing for operations and an increasing number of men and women suffering from raised blood pressure and cholesterol.

It is amazing how many times I receive emails that ask questions about nutrition but end up asking about how to spice up sex lives. Most people assume that it is their age to blame for lack lustre performances and this applies to both men and women. However, they are only partly correct; as there is no doubt that both sexes suffer from a reduction in the sex hormones and an imbalance for a period of time that will affect sex drive and performance.

The quick answer according to the many emails that I receive and the media coverage is to buy a "little blue pill" and keep going for four hours or more!

That is all very well but if you are a middle aged man or woman for that matter, who embarks on this course of action, you should be aware of the real dangers involved, particularly if you buy from unknown sources on the Internet.

Sexual performance should be pleasurable and satisfying into our 80's and 90's. I am not a sex therapist so if the problem is boredom or poor self image then you will need to buy another book. Although having said that, you should feel considerably better about your self image when you are a healthy weight and have a great deal more energy than currently.

However, I am pretty certain that the secret to achieving a long and healthy sex life does not start with taking the "little blue pill" but begins in the kitchen! Hence the carrot!

Your body's health is dependent on the nutrients in the food that you eat. Lousy diet results in poor health and low energy. Everything that you put in your mouth is processed by the body and used to produce the chemical reactions required for not only our everyday functions but also our sex drive. You put contaminated fuel into the system and your body will be unable to fire on all cylinders.

What this book offers is not the quick fix you may be looking for in time for this evening but it could well improve and spice up your sex life in a short space of time and for the long term.

In our heads and hearts we remain at an age when we were slim, young and raring to go. Unfortunately our modern lifestyle has created a body that cannot keep up with our self imposed expectations.

It takes two to tango and if you are in a relationship then both of you should read this guide to a healthy middle age. It is not only men who are suffering the effects of modern day stresses and diet and the programmes in the second half of the book will be of as much benefit to men and women equally.

Before you decide that perhaps this longer term approach is not for you it might be an idea to answer the questionnaire over the page and reassess not just your sexual health but the health and longevity of your entire body.

1. Questionnaire

If you answer yes to most of the following questions your sex life is at risk.

- Are you more than 2 stone, 28 lbs or 12 kilos overweight?
- Do you participate in less than 2 hours regular exercise per week?
- Do you eat less than six portions of fresh fruit and vegetables per day?
- Do you eat fried food more than three times per week?
- Do you eat processed prepared meals more than twice a week?
- Do you eat white bread, pasta and rice?
- Do you drink less than 2 litres of fluid per day?
- Do you suffer from high blood pressure?
- Do you take high blood pressure medication?
- Do you suffer from elevated cholesterol levels?
- Do you take medication for cholesterol?
- Do you suffer from elevated blood sugar levels or diabetes?
- Do you take medication for diabetes?
- Do you drink more than two units of alcohol per day?
- Do you smoke?
- Do you suffer from depression?
- Do you take medication for depression?
- Do you have a heart condition such as angina?
- Do you take heart medication?
- Do you have an enlarged prostate and take medication?
- Have you been diagnosed with vascular disease?

2. Why not Take Viagra?

That is a very good question. You have erectile dysfunction, you want to enjoy an active sex life and all you have to do is to take a 'little blue pill' and all will be wonderful ... or so the advertisements and spam email would have you believe!

I have suffered anaphylactic shock three times in my life and nearly died. Two of those were from medication prescribed to me. On other occasions I have reacted sufficiently badly to a drug that I have been unable to take them ever again. These included the contraceptive pill, penicillin and aspirin.

How many of you are prescribed medication or buy a packet of pills over the counter and sit down with the small print and find out just what this pill might do to you? Everything that is put into your body has to be processed and is added to the already complex mixture of chemicals and fluids within your system. Your major organs including your brain, kidneys and liver will be affected to one degree or another and if you are unlucky enough to be the small percentage of people who reacts badly to this particular drug then it could be fatal.

So, What Do We Know About Viagra?

1. *Firstly, Viagra was NOT designed as a cure for erectile dysfunction. It is a treatment for another disease.*

Viagra first hit the news in 1998 and since then has been taken by millions of older men who wanted to recapture the potency of their youth despite the fact that many were not really suffering any form of sexual dysfunction, simply the natural reduction in male hormones that takes place in middle age and the side affect of poor lifestyle choices. It was thought by many to be an aphrodisiac and a magical way to produce the perfect sex life. *Wrong.* An enjoyable sex life for both people in a relationship is so much more than a four hour erection.

2. *The drug was originally developed for men who suffered from chest pains.*

The original pill contained *sildenafil citrate* and it is interesting to note that due to some severe and fatal reactions it was not prescribed for men who suffered the following.

- Heart disease
- Glaucoma
- High Blood Pressure
- Diabetes
- Patients taking nitrates for heart disease.

Three of these contraindications are for physical problems that contribute to erectile dysfunction in the first place!

Some research indicated that sildenafil citrate might have properties that would help treat erectile dysfunction and a number of clinical studies were conducted which showed that Viagra could produce and sustain an erection under varied circumstances.

The active ingredient in Viagra is nitric oxide which increases the levels of an enzyme which in turn relaxes muscles in the corpus cavernosum, the sponge like areas of the penis. This expands to allow blood to fill the area resulting in an erection.

It only took six months to bring the drug to market which is a very short period of time and the issue of side effects or outside consultation with experts was not included in the data.

There are at least two clinical studies that have shown that sildenafil might cause sudden blindness and other vision problems.

Newer impotency drugs have also been associated with vision problems. This is caused by 'non-arteritic ischemic optic neuropathy' where the blood supply is reduced to the optic nerve causing permanent nerve damage.

The FDA did publish guidelines for the prescription of the drug which was valid when it was in the hands of doctors but has become largely redundant now that you can buy Viagra or one of the more recent, and largely untested drugs, over the Internet.

You can be sure that the spammers are not going to tell you that you should not take the drug if you are already taking nitrates for heart disease.

- If you suffer from angina, where the blood vessels of the heart are narrowed, the mix of Viagra and nitrates can reduce your blood pressure to dangerously low levels. Any prolonged reduction in blood pressure decreases the blood flow and deprives the heart of blood leading to a heart attack.
- If you have a blood disorder such as leukaemia you should not take Viagra or similar drugs.
- If you have an unusually shaped penis you should not take Viagra or similar drugs.
- Any of your current medications, including over the counter products, could cause an adverse reaction with Viagra or similar drug.
- It is potentially dangerous to take a combination of ED drugs.

Side Effects of Taking Viagra

The problem with side effects is that we only know about the ones that the pharmaceutical companies feel they should share with us. I realise that this sounds very cynical but if you consider that the vast majority of research trials are not only funded but run by the pharmaceutical companies themselves, then it really does not lead to much confidence in the findings. If you take a million men who are taking Viagra and were to ask them to call in and report any of the following side effects anonymously I believe you might have a vastly different picture as to the frequency of the short and long term effects of taking the drug.

These are the side effects that they have been willing to share with us and we are assured that they only occur in a small percentage of men taking Viagra.

- Headaches
- Flushing
- Indigestion
- Nasal congestion
- Urinary tract infection
- Mild and temporary vision changes
- Diarrhoea
- Dizziness
- Rash
- Respiratory tract infections
- Back Pain symptoms.
- Flu

What is more interesting, as we look at some of the other medications that middle aged men are now encouraged to take for their lifestyle related conditions such as high blood pressure and elevated cholesterol, is that the combination of the side effects make a possibly fatal cocktail.

I was interested to read about any fatalities from taking Viagra and again these are only statistics that have been verified as caused by the drug. Like MRSA the figures are probably understated as the causes could well be attributed to other factors such as age, smoking or diet. You wonder how many of the deceased even admitted that they took Viagra in the first place. I am sure that many doctors are unaware that their patients are taking Viagra or a similar sex enhancer that they have bought over the Internet and should they die suddenly from a stroke or a heart attack it may not be the first question that comes to mind unless they die with an unexplained erection.

If you check the Internet medical sites that give statistics for specific drugs it makes for interesting reading. According to findings published in July 2013 based on FDA reports, 1,028 deaths have been attributed to taking Viagra, which is just one of the brands available, and does not include those that are purchased over the Internet for which there are no figures. Side effects that have been reported are surprising. Out of 32,500 who reported side effects nearly 9,000 males, mainly over 60 years of age, found the drug ineffective, almost 4,000 experienced sexual dysfunction and 3,000 experienced impotence. The rest of the side effects ranged from headaches and chest pains and also includes the 1,028 who died.

These deaths are difficult to attribute entirely to taking the medication because of underlying existing health issues or because of interactions with other drugs being taken. Most worrying are the deaths where there appear to be no cause in otherwise healthy individuals.

These figures relate to patients who had been prescribed the medication, so what about the millions of men worldwide who are buying through the Internet without being examined by a doctor? How many of *their* deaths have been attributed to taking a sexual enhancer?

So we have now established that, as far as the pharmaceutical companies are concerned, the drug is safe. We have also determined that it is not a cure for erectile dysfunction but a treatment.

Its main appeal is that it is fast acting, relatively cheap and can be bought freely without prescription – if you are willing to take the risk.

What I am proposing is not necessarily fast acting although you should feel the benefits to your overall health in a relatively short space of time. Some of the lifestyle changes I am suggesting you make will of course involve some deprivation. You will be reducing your alcohol content and if you are still smoking then giving that up will save you a small fortune. The good news is that both these harmful habits can cause problems with sexual performance, not only on the night but systematically over the years through vascular damage and toxic build up.

The programme at the back of the book is one that you can follow for the rest of your life. The cost of the book has to be taken into account of course, but it would be good to think that those of you who choose to read, digest and follow the programme could end up with normal blood pressure, cholesterol and blood sugar levels and off medication for the rest of your lives – not only that you will save yourself about £1 a "little blue pill"

As a reminder: please do not suddenly stop taking any prescribed medication. Talk to your doctor and tell him that you would like to monitor your progress over the next six months and with his help, and with positive changes to your diet and lifestyle, you would like to be drug free.

So ... *Forget the Viagra and reach for the carrots!*

Summary

- We are our own worst enemies and spend most of our lives making poor lifestyle choices that only impact us in middle age.
- It is never too late to change and even into our 70s and 80s eating a healthy diet and giving up smoking and excessive alcohol consumption can change our sex lives.
- There are side-effects to all drugs that are ingested into our finely balanced operating system and if our body is already in overwhelm due to our poor diet and lifestyle our major organs may be affected more severely.
- Our bodies are our only asset and if we want them to last a lifetime and also enjoy a high quality of life including a

healthy sex drive we need to take care of it and that means eating the right foods.
- Sex is not just a physical act although in our youth it would appear so. It is also an emotional and mental activity and feeling good about your body and what you see in the mirror is part of the process.

3. If You Don't Know How It Works, How Can You Fix It?

It is not my intention to write a medical encyclopaedia but I found that the only way that I could successfully learn about nutrition was to understand how the body uses nutrition to operate. I could not design an individual eating programme for a client with obesity, high blood pressure and elevated cholesterol if I did not understand why he was suffering from those conditions in the first place. When I was facing a personal health crisis I had to change not just my lifestyle but certain habits of a lifetime. Apart from biology classes and an 'O' Level in the science, I had learnt nothing further about my body until my early 40s. Being 330 lbs with its attendant health problems focuses your mind somewhat and having spent a lifetime of listening to others who I thought knew better, I decided to find out for myself.

I developed a fascination with the human body and its wonderful complex machinery. I appreciate it now in a way I never could before, despite the fact that my own is far from the stereotype of the 'perfect' body, at 60 years old I no longer have life threatening conditions that I was told would end my life in my mid 40s.

Just remember your body is your greatest asset and the only one you are going to get in this lifetime. You should be taking care of it in the same way as you do any other precious asset, your family, your house or your bank account!

To understand why you might be suffering from erectile dysfunction (ED) or any other related sexual problem then first you need to find out the basics of the organs that are not working efficiently.

Like most of the complicated operations within our bodies it is easy to take the reproductive system for granted. For women, the way it works is a little more obvious with several monthly indicators that let us know how well it is functioning or how badly.

With men, provided there is no pain associated with the normal functions of peeing or having sex it is easy to forget the intricacies of the chemical and physical activities behind the act.

It is important that all of us have an understanding of how our bodies work as a whole, because spare parts are in short supply. We demand that our body lasts us a lifetime but the way our body is treated from birth has a direct impact on our health as children, teenagers, young adults, middle age and old age. The food that we put in our mouths as a child and young adult will affect your chances of suffering from high blood pressure, elevated cholesterol and diabetes in middle age, all of which are contributory causes to sexual dysfunction in both men and women. Even worse is that the drugs used to treat these conditions are likely to be the causes of lowered libido and sexual performance.

Add in being overweight, arterial disease, heart problems and impaired immune system and you have the perfect environment for a poor general quality of life, let alone sex life.

It is as important for women to understand the male reproductive system as their own. I have worked with young women who were desperate to start a baby and who were eager and willing to follow any healthy programme that put their bodies in the best possible health to conceive. Trouble is when asked about their partner's lifestyles they did not seem to realise that it made any difference. They only have to provide the sperm, don't they? Wrong, like any substance within our bodies, sperm is the product of our diet and lifestyle and if they are too weak to swim up through the labyrinth of the female reproductive system then conception is not going to happen.

It is important that you understand how your reproductive system works and can share that knowledge with your partner. In following chapters I am going to focus on some of the contributory factors to erectile dysfunction but it is important that your partner understands these factors as well, as a knowledgeable and supportive partner is essential in managing this condition.

Summary

- Knowing how your body works even on a basic level helps you understand where the process might have gone wrong.
- It takes two to tango and it is important that both partners are aware of how each other's sexual and reproductive systems work.
- If your body is tired, full of prescription medication and you are missing all the essential nutrients necessary for a fully functioning, hormonally rich reproductive system, then getting an erection may be the last thing on your brain's agenda. Survival is.

4. The Brain

Most of my clients laugh like a drain when I tell them that actually it is all in the mind! Sexuality is a combination of factors and the laws of attraction have been researched for thousands of years to try and come up with the perfect equation. However, the brain plays a very important role in our sex lives and if your brain is not functioning as well as it might then other parts of your body will be affected. Your hormones do not just appear in the body from nowhere – they are directed by a master controller in the brain and although the response is automatic it can be affected by localised conditions. So I have chosen to start by taking a look at this amazingly complex organ which is still largely a mystery to scientists because taking care of your brain health can not only help your sex life but also your mental and physical health into old age.

The Basics

For me, the brain has always been a fascinating part of the body as it is this organ rather than our hearts that makes us the person we are.

It is the evolution of this organ which has distinguished us from all other living creatures. As we continue to pollute this world of ours I expect that it will be the brain which will be our main survival tool. It will be brain power that hopefully finds solutions for climate changes, the deteriorating ozone layer and the increasingly worrying problem of where we will all live. It will take the combined brain power of many people to find us that place in space that may have to be our new home. All the advances in science and medicine are made possible by the workings of this powerful organ and taking care of it should be our number one priority.

Much of this activity is in the future and in other hands. We are in the here and now and facing enough challenges of our own. One of them being how to keep our own bodies fit, healthy and functioning to a ripe old age. How wonderful to be able to look back at a lifetime of 90 or 100 years and remember every minute of it, every person we have ever met and every experience we have enjoyed. It is possible, but if the current trend of eating processed foods with poor nutritional value increases, we will begin to diminish our brain power and risk ending our lives not even remembering our own names.

In this chapter you will also find information on Alzheimer's disease. As we look at the brain, and the effects of damage on the various parts of the organ, you will begin to see where some of the symptoms of Alzheimer's originate. Apart from direct trauma to the brain, resulting in long term damage, or genetic risk factors, there is the more probable damage sustained by brain cell death due to nutritional deficiency or the effects of a stroke. Both of these conditions are directly affected by our lifestyle choices and diet.

The Anatomy of the Brain

First we need to understand the anatomy of the brain and how the various parts affect who we are and our abilities to function everyday.

Protected within the bony and tough skull, the brain is an organ of many parts. Each part works independently of the others but with a common purpose. There are excellent communication channels between each half of the brain and each functioning unit and this provides us with a seamless operation that enables us to see, breathe, think, smell, eat, process food, make love, talk and move amongst other things without really thinking about it.

The Brain Stem

This is the lower extension of the brain where it connects to the spinal cord. This is the survival centre of the brain and the Medulla Oblongata at the base of the brain-stem governs breathing, digestion, heart rate, blood pressure and our ability to be awake and alert. Most of the cranial nerves are from the brain-stem, which is the pathway for all the fibre tracts passing up and down from the peripheral nerves and spinal cord to the highest parts of the brain.

The Cerebral Cortex

The outermost layer of the cerebral hemisphere which is composed of grey matter. There are two hemispheres that are asymmetrical

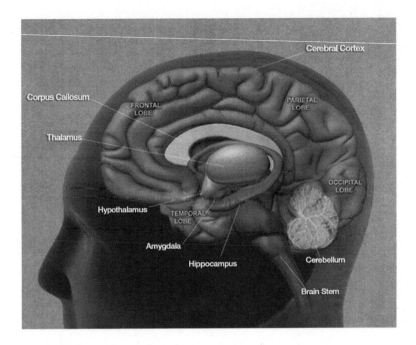

Drawing of the human brain, showing important structures
Public Domain photo courtesy of National Institute for Aging,
a branch of NIH. http://www.nia.nih.gov

and both are able to analyse sensory data, perform memory functions, learn new information, form thoughts and make decisions. The two hemispheres however have different abilities. The left hemisphere is the serious side of our brain that can interpret information, do mathematics, learn language and reason. The right hemisphere is more the fun side of the brain able to process an amazing amount of sensory input in seconds to provide a complete picture of the immediate environment. This side also governs functions such as dancing or complicated movements and we also store our visual and auditory memories here.

The Corpus Callosum

This connects the two hemispheres to allow them to communicate with each other. This is essential if we for example want to combine the two individual abilities into one. Taking a complicated language such as music and playing it on an instrument for example would require co-ordination between the two sides of the brain.

The two hemispheres have different lobes and the Frontal lobes are for reasoning and memory. At the front of these lobes you will find the Prefrontal areas, which determine our ability to concentrate, reason and elaborate on information. They also are sometimes called the Gatekeeper of the brain as they govern our judgement and our inhibitions. Our personality and emotional traits are also sited here as well as our movement capabilities and language skills. Damage to the frontal lobes may result in loss of recent memory, confusion, inability to concentrate, difficulty in taking in new information and behavioural disorders.

The Parietal Lobes

These are located behind the frontal lobes at the top of the brain and again have different duties within the scope of the brain. The right lobe enables us to find our way around spaces both those we are familiar with and new ones that we encounter. The left lobe enables our ability to understand spoken and written language.

The Parietal lobes also contain the primary sensory cortex, which controls sensation, or touch pressure and behind this cortex is an area which controls finer sensations such as texture, weight, size and shape. Damage to this part of the brain can leave a person unable to discriminate between the various sensory stimuli or to be able to locate and recognise parts of their own body. They may also lose the ability to translate the speech into the written word.

The Occipital Lobes

These are right at the back of the brain and they process visual information and not only are these lobes responsible for visual reception but they also contain association areas that help us recognise shapes and colours. Damage to this area will affect the sight.

The Temporal Lobes

These are on each side of the brain about level with the ears. These lobes allow us to tell one smell from another and one sound from another. They also help in sorting new information and are believed to be responsible for short-term memory. Again the two separate lobes have different responsibilities. The right lobe is mainly involved in visual memory such as pictures or faces and the left lobe remembers words and names. Damage to this part of the brain may result in loss of hearing, panic and behavioural problems.

Within the brain is the Limbic system, which contains our smell pathways and also some very important glands that affect our sex drive, anger and fear mechanisms and our emotions. These pathways are of vital importance to the efficient running of our operational systems within the bodies and the health of these glands and pathways will have an impact on our general health and longevity. Damage to this part of the brain can result in a loss of the sense of smell, agitation, loss of control of emotions and loss of recent memory.

How can we keep all the parts of our brain healthy and functioning for an entire lifetime?

Like all our other major organs, the brain requires a complex combination of oxygen and nutrients to sustain, nourish, repair and renew itself. Apart from eating a healthy diet, the nutrients need to get access to the brain and there are only a couple of options. The main arterial route into the brain, taking oxygen rich blood with the necessary nutrients is the Carotid Artery.

Carotid Artery

Like all arteries that supply blood to the various parts of the body such as the heart and brain, the carotid arteries can also develop a build-up of fat and cholesterol deposits, called plaque, on the inside. Over time this layer of plaque increases, hardening and blocking the arteries. This means that the oxygen and nutrients that your brain needs to function are very restricted.

Unfortunately the knock-on effect of a narrowed artery is that plaque can break off and travel to the smaller arteries in the brain, blocking those pathways. Additionally, a blood clot can form and because the arteries have become so narrow it cannot pass and causes a blockage. This is what leads to a stroke.

Later in the book I have devoted a chapter to Cholesterol and how you can achieve a normal level with the correct balance of good and bad cholesterol.

Alzeimer's Disease

If I were to put my greatest fear into words, it would not be that I become wrinkled and physically decrepit but that I would forget everything of importance in my life. I have presented two or three programmes on the radio on the subject and it has always resulted in e-mails and telephone calls from listeners who have the same fears about age related dementia.

Dementia is actually a collective name for progressive degenerative brain diseases, which affect our memory, thought, behaviour and emotions. It is not a normal result of ageing and it does not seem to have any specific social, economic, ethnic or geographical links. It can affect different people in different ways, which makes it difficult sometimes to diagnose and to treat. There is no known cure, but there are ways that we can modify our lifestyle to reduce our risks of brain degeneration and to slow down any process that has already begun.

Effects of the Disease

Alzheimer's disease is the most common form of dementia and accounts for around 60% of all cases. The disease is degenerative over a period of years and destroys brain cells and nerve cells causing a disruption to the transmitters, which carry messages in the brain, particularly those that are responsible for our memories.

As the disease progresses, the brain shrinks and gaps develop in the temporal lobe and hippocampus. These areas are responsible for storing and retrieving new information. The damage results in a reduction in a person's ability to remember events that happened in the short term, to speak, think and to make decisions. All this is both frightening and confusing, as a person will be aware of these lapses in the early stages of the condition.

What are the Symptoms of Alzheimer's?

In the beginning, there may be infrequent lapses in memory, forgetting where keys have been left or perhaps failing to switch off electric cookers or other equipment. A person will start to forget the names of everyday objects or people that they are usually very familiar with. They can also suffer from mood swings and panic attacks.

As the disease progresses these symptoms worsen and there is an element of confusion over completing every day tasks such as shopping, cooking and more dangerously driving.

The changes in personality are often attributable to fear and the awareness that something is very wrong. In the earlier stages people tend to try and hide the symptoms. This happens because, much of the time, they will be aware that there is a problem and will not want to accept that this could be as serious a problem as dementia.

In the advanced stages it is not only extremely stressful for the person concerned but also very distressing for their immediate family. We have experience of the problem with a close family friend who was in his 80's and was looking after his wife who had Alzheimer's for two years before she went into a home. At that point he was no longer able to cope. She was in danger of hurting herself as she was wandering off in the middle of the night, falling over and hurting herself as well as becoming terrified and disorientated.

What are the Risk Factors?

It is difficult to pinpoint the exact cause of dementia, but there are several probable links that have been the subject of research in recent years.

There is some evidence of a genetic link to the disease, but that is not proven. Lifestyle most definitely will have played a contributory role as exposure to toxins from smoking, excessive alcohol consumption or work environment will cause damage to the body as a whole and certainly to the brain. There is obviously natural age related degeneration of the entire body and its systems to take into account and any previous head trauma may be part of the problem. There are links to chemical contamination including poisoning from mercury – which can be found in some of the fish that we eat – and also from aluminium, which is most commonly linked to the metal in some of our cooking utensils.

Some recent statistics suggest that at least 10% of those over 65 and 50% of those over 85 years old will be suffering from varying degrees of dementia. We unfortunately have no control over natural ageing, or our genetic background, which means that we should be looking at ways to prevent or minimise the risk of us developing the disease from a much earlier age than our 60's.

The incidence of a genetic cause of Alzheimer's disease is minimal. Exposure to toxins and poor diet is a more likely cause, for two very good reasons. As a person ages, all the systems run down and this includes the digestive systems that metabolise food for its nutrients. Coupled with the fact that older people tend to lose their appetite, nutrients are in short supply, unless supplemented. Also, the ability to eliminate toxins is equally sluggish allowing a harmful build up of damaging substances in the tissues of the body, including the brain.

What is interesting however is the possibility of a bacterial connection to dementia. Chlamydia Pneumoniae is a common airborne bacterium that infects as many as 70% of the World's population and there is research that suggests that there is a link to bacteria and brain disease. This would make sense, as the immune system would also be repressed along with other systems in an elderly person's body, leaving them wide open to infections and probable cell damage

Diet for the Brain

The healthy eating plan for life at the back of the book is designed to help your body achieve healthy cholesterol levels. It will also provide the essential nutrients that the brain requires to function healthily and efficiently.

Some Things to Think About

If you currently take in a great deal of saturated or hydrogenated fats in your diet you need to look at some of your other risk factors. If you are a heavy smoker or already suffer from high blood pressure it is time to take a look at your lifestyle as a whole. A good start would be to reduce your intake of foods that are high in saturated fats from animal food sources and also hydrogenated fats found in processed foods.

Good Things to Do

- Reduce input of animal fats & hydrogenated fats
- Substitute with olive oil or sunflower oil
- Avoid frying foods
- Increase intake of fruit & vegetables
- Eat raw fruit & vegetables where possible
- Eat oats & brown rice
- Get more Omega-3 fatty acids – oily fish
- Eat more nuts – but beware of the calories

You will find more details in the Chapter on Cholesterol.

Summary

- The brain needs a healthy balanced diet to function efficiently and to prevent degenerative diseases
- High blood pressure and cholesterol levels will affect the health of your brain.
- Your erection may be the result of physical stimulation but your brain also needs to be engaged in the process. If your master controller is on the blink so is your sex life.
- Your brain cannot be replaced – as yet we cannot transplant a new one in when the old one fails. Feed it well and use it or lose it.
- Get in the habit of thinking about what you are putting in your mouth and the affect it will have on your brain.

Research Notes

Researches from the University of Navarra, Spain, published findings online in the *Journal of Neurology, Neurosurgery and Psychiatry* on a long term study on the impact of a Mediterranean diet on brain power. 522 men and women between the ages of 55 and 80 who were all considered to have risk factors associated with heart disease, diabetes and family history, were divided into three groups that consumed olive oil, mixed nuts or the recommended low-fat heart diet.

After six years, those on the olive oil and the nuts as whole scored higher in the mental exercises than those on the low fat diet. Of the 35 who did eventually develop dementia 17 were on the low fat diet, 12 on the olive oil and 6 on the nuts.

A small study at Maryland University in the United States published results in the *Journal of Alzeimer's Disease* which indicated that moderate exercise in a small group of 60 to 88 year olds with mild brain impairment showed both physical and mental improvements. It is believed that the reduced stress resulting from the exercise enabled the participants to think more clearly. The study has encouraged the researchers to continue to confirm the results and to determine long term effects of exercise on brain function.

5. The Male Reproductive System

The male reproductive system produces and releases semen into the reproductive system of the female during sexual intercourse with the aim of fertilising one or more of her eggs. It is also responsible for maturing a boy to manhood at puberty at around 10 to 14 years old.

As with women, men's reproductive organs are divided into two parts, the internal and external organs and the gonads called the testes. When boys reach puberty, gonadotropic hormones are secreted by the pituitary gland and the gonads grow and become active. The gonadotropic hormones also stimulate the production of the androgens or testosterone hormones, which in turn will promote the growth, and development of external genitalia as well as stimulating changes in the larynx. One of the outward signs of a boy reaching puberty is his voice breaking and then becoming deeper over the next few months.

The male reproductive organs (*refer to the diagram on the next page*) are external and internal and include the testicles; duct system made up of the epididymis and vas deferens, the spermatic cord, the seminal vesicles and the penis.

The testicles or testes are oval shaped and grow to about 2 inches (5 centimetres) in length and 1 inch (3 centimetres) in width. They are formed in the embryo from a ridge of tissue at the back of the abdomen. They gradually move down the abdomen during the pregnancy reaching the scrotum in time for the birth. They consist of seminiferous tubules where sperm is manufactured and interstitial cells which produce the testosterone hormone. As a boy matures he produces more and more testosterone and in addition to his deepening voice he will develop more body hair, bigger muscles and produce sperm.

Alongside the testes are the epididymis and the vas deferens of the male duct system. The epididymis consists of elaborately

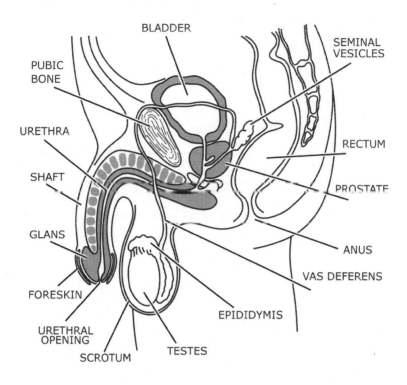

BLADDER

SEMINAL
VESICLES

PUBIC
BONE

URETHRA

RECTUM

SHAFT

PROSTATE

GLANS

ANUS

VAS DEFERENS

FORESKIN

EPIDIDYMIS

URETHRAL
OPENING

TESTES

SCROTUM

Male Reproductive Organs

coiled tubes that are attached to the back of each testis. These carry the sperm into the vas deferens, an extension of the epididymis that has become a muscular tube that takes the sperm up into the penis in semen.

The testes and the duct system are protected by a skin bag called the scrotum. One of its main roles is to maintain a slightly lower temperature than the rest of the body otherwise the testes will be unable to produce sperm.

There is a complex connective system between the penis and the testes called the spermatic cord that not only suspends the testes but contains and protects the blood vessels, sperm and hormone carrying tubes, nerves and lymph system that supply the scrotum. It is also covered by a number of layers including the cremasteric muscle, which is responsible for contracting the scrotum in extremes of temperature or during ejaculation.

As the sperm move up the vas deferens they pause in a storage area called the ampulla where they are bathed in seminal fluid from the vesicles situated just above each side of the prostate gland. This fluid stimulates the sperm to move spontaneously and actively as it passes through the prostate gland and penis into the vagina.

The prostate gland is a very small walnut shaped structure that sits at the base of the bladder and surrounds the ejaculatory ducts at the base of the urethra. Its role is to produce an alkaline fluid that mixes with the semen from the vesicles before it is passed into the penis to be ejaculated. This probably acts as a booster for the sperm keeping them active and therefore more likely to fertilise an egg should the opportunity arise. Unfortunately problems with the prostate can arise as men age and this either results in difficulties with the bladder or actual disease of the prostate.

The shaft of the penis contains a central tube called the urethra leading to a small hole in the head of the penis called the meatus. This enables urine to pass from the bladder and out of the body or allows for the ejaculation of semen during intercourse. Because the urethra has a dual purpose, a strong muscle ring at the connection between the bladder and the tube ensures that urine only passes through when intended.

The penis is made up of groups of tissue that are responsible for erections. There is a complex interaction between the blood vessels and the nervous system following sexual arousal. Desire can be stimulated by a number of factors, some of which are unique to the individual, but usually include our sensory organs and our imagination which is complimented by physical stimulation of the penis. The rich network of blood vessels in the penis becomes distended when a man is aroused. The blood is unable to flow back into the body and the penis therefore stiffens and rises as the internal pressure increases. After ejaculation the blood flow reduces to normal levels and the penis returns to a flaccid state.

All boys are born with a fold of skin that protects the glans from injury. This is called the foreskin and during an erection this peels back to allow the tip to be stimulated during intercourse. A lubricant called smegma is produced by the foreskin and the skin on the glans to make this action smooth, but poor hygiene, or irritants can lead to severe infections. Circumcision is often carried out on baby boys for both religious and health reasons.

6. Disorders of the Male Reproductive System

Although this book is primarily about sexual dysfunction in older men it is important for any younger readers to understand that many of the causes of male infertility are also causes of sexual dysfunction in later life. Male infertility can also respond positively to changes in diet and lifestyle and once those changes have been made and are maintained over a lifetime the chances are that erectile dysfunction will not even occur.

As with later life problems with our sex lives in both men and women, occupational, environmental and recreational factors play an enormous role. Some of these include high levels of stress; disturbances in the sleep cycle, drugs, smoking, excessive alcohol intake, toxins and chemical exposure at work or in the home environment and all will effect the production and health of sperm as well as sexual performance in general.

Fertility and sexual performance in men requires normal functioning of the hypothalamus, pituitary gland, and testes. Therefore, a variety of different conditions can lead to problems with the reproductive system. It is believed that 40% to 50% of infertility problems have no identifiable cause. This number may well apply to functional problems with the sex organs as well. This is where lifestyle and diet may play a major role in helping overcome the problems.

Effects of Drugs and Alcohol

Studies into the affect of alcohol on erectile dysfunction are mixed but there still seems to be a strong indication that moderate intake of around 2 to 3 units a night will increase sexual desire but reduce sexual performance.

Effects of Smoking

Smoking decreases sex drive and therefore frequency of sexual encounters. Vascular disease caused by smoking will affect a man's ability to achieve and sustain an erection.

Malnutrition and Obesity

I have often informed a very overweight client that they are suffering from malnutrition which is usually met with caustic laughter. But in fact today's obesity problems are not due to high calorie intake but low nutritional content of those calories. People are eating rubbish and the body is not getting what it needs to function properly. Therefore they are suffering from malnutrition.

Certainly with sexual dysfunction there is a link between malnutrition and poor hormone production, which I will look at later, as it is my opinion that diet is one of the leading contributory factors when we look at sexual performance in older men.

Exposure to Toxins, Chemicals and Infections

Exposure to external pollutants or internal infections can not only damage parts of the male reproductive system such as the testes but also disrupt the normal hormonal function of the relevant glands. There is increasing evidence that our modern world is responsible for a worldwide decline in male fertility and it is likely that as exposure affects hormone production it will also affect sexual performance as we age.

Pesticides containing oestrogen-like chemicals are widely thought to be responsible for the increase in testicular and prostate cancers. Over exposure to oestrogen in males results in a reduction of the Sertolli cells (necessary for the initial development of sperm).

Hydrocarbons and other industrial compounds have been shown to affect the sperm count of workers in rubber factories and petrochemical plants. Combine this level of exposure to cigarette smoking and the risk of infertility increases significantly and therefore may also contribute to dysfunction sexually.

Radiation treatments and X-rays affect any rapidly dividing cells so sperm cells are vulnerable to damage. It may take up to 2 years after radiation treatment for normal sperm production and in some cases it may never recover.

Something as commonplace as a laptop computer may affect a man's fertility if he is accustomed to working with it actually on his lap. Testicles need to be at a cooler temperature than the body which is why they are outside in the first place. The computer will raise the temperature of the testicles sufficiently to affect sperm production.

After surgery or radiation treatment for cancer of the prostate there is a high probability of impotence. After surgery impotence occurs right away but may improve over a number of months or years. With radiation the impotence may not happen immediately but develop over a period of a year or more. They estimate that 75% of men will be impotent within 5 years of radiation treatment if they experienced some problems before and about half the men who had normal erection before treatment become impotent in the same time frame.

If this is the case, and you are recovering from prostate surgery or radiation treatment, then please work with your doctor in regard to your impotence. Provided you do not have heart problems or are on any medication that might interact with drugs such as Viagra then they may be appropriate.

However, even if this is the case, the programme at the back of the book will certainly do you no harm as it should improve your general health including any blood pressure, cholesterol or blood sugar issues you are also contending with which might prohibit the use of sexual enhancing drugs.

A healthy body is also less likely to host cancerous cells and keeping your body free of this disease is your priority.

Hormonal Deficiencies

Gonadotropine releasing hormone (GnRH) is the primary hormone that stimulates the process that leads to the release of testosterone and other reproductive hormones. Low levels of testosterone will result in a lower sex drive and performance. It is natural in both men and women to experience a reduction in these sex hormones in our 40's and 50's but they should not signal the end of an active sex life. But, combine the reduction in these hormones with lifestyle factors and your body will not be able to function as it once did.

Later I will be taking a close look at cholesterol and the medication currently used to treat abnormalities. Cholesterol is a precursor for many of the hormones in the body relating to our sexuality and if it is reduced dramatically following medication it can lead to a corresponding reduction in testosterone and other sexual hormones at a time of your life when you need all you can produce.

Testosterone

Testosterone is the most important of the male sex hormones called androgens.

It is responsible for the development of the male sexual and reproductive organs that I have already covered earlier on the male reproductive system.

It also stimulates the development of the secondary male sex characteristics such as an increase in muscle mass, increased body and facial hair, enlargement of the larynx and the vocal chord thickening, which leads to a deepening of the voice.

The testes produce the testosterone regulated by a complex chain of messages that begin in the hypothalamus in the brain. The hypothalamus secretes Gonadotropine-releasing hormone (GnRH) to the pituitary gland in carefully timed bursts. This triggers the release of leutenising hormone (LH) which in turn stimulates the Lydia cells of the testes to produce testosterone. At puberty the production of testosterone increases very rapidly and declines equally rapidly after the age of 50. This change in testosterone levels is one of the reasons that it is quite likely that men will suffer some form of menopause and therefore reduction in sexual performance and they need to ensure that their diet reflects the reduction in this bone and muscle-protecting hormone. It is not only our sexual performance which suffers but also the strength of our skeleton, joints and muscles, so eating the right foods are critical at this stage in our lives.

The testes produce between 4 mg and 7 mg of testosterone per day but like the two female hormones oestrogen and progesterone this decreases naturally with age. There are rare cases where young boys fail to develop at puberty causing problems with bone and muscle development and underdeveloped sexual organs. The likely cause is damage to the hypothalamus, pituitary gland or the testes themselves.

Problems With the Penis

A reduction in hormones and poor lifestyle are just some of the reasons why a man might experience lack of sex drive or poor erectile function. No one penis is the same and because it is an external organ it is subject to damage and also to infections that will affect its ability to achieve an erection.

There are a number of physical reasons for abnormalities in the penis and some are evident at birth or very shortly afterwards.

There are some cases of babies being born with ambiguous genitalia with no clear indication if it is a boy or a girl. In some cases a baby boy may have a very small or non-existent penis but have some testicular tissue present. In other cases a baby may have both testicular and ovarian tissue. Surgery is usually carried out when appropriate or hormonal treatment given to the child as it develops. It obviously carries not only physical implications but emotional and mental trauma that needs to be addressed as the child grows towards puberty.

Hypospadias is a condition where the urethra opens on the underside of the penis instead of the tip. It actually is quite common occurring in between 1 in 150–300 babies born and there is a strong genetic link to the problem. It is caused by the urethra failing to develop in the foetus to the correct length and it is usually corrected by surgery when the baby is between 6 and 12 months old. Babies with this problem cannot be circumcised until the problem is corrected.

Phimosis results in a tightness of the foreskin of the penis and is quite common in new born and young boys. It usually resolves itself but if it interferes with urination then circumcision is performed.

There are a number of medical problems associated with the penis. Two of the more common conditions amongst uncircumcised males are the possible infection of the glans or head of the penis called Balanitis or inflammation of the foreskin called Posthitis. They are usually caused by either a bacterial or yeast infection and from a very young age boys should be taught about hygiene and how to keep areas under the foreskin clean.

If a boy or young man is sexually active and not using condoms then he is at risk of contracting a sexually transmitted disease. Genital warts and Chlamydia have long term effects on the reproductive system of both girls and boys and it is extremely important that they understand the implications of having unprotected sex. Unfortunately, recent studies are indicating that a large majority of teenagers know about the dangers but choose to ignore them. This is very sad as most will wonder in their late twenties and early thirties why they are unable to have children themselves. In our modern world sexually transmitted diseases are on the increase rather than decline and include Syphilis, Gonorrhoea, Hepatitis B and AIDS.

Prostate Problems

In a young man the prostate is about the size of a walnut and it slowly gets larger as a man matures. If it gets too large however it can begin to cause problems with the urinary tract resulting in frequent urination and in some cases discomfort as well as impotence.

This is called benign prostatic hyperplasia (BPH) and is very common in men over 60 years old. If problems with urination occur especially at night then a doctor should be consulted. Usually a rectal examination or scans will detect the enlarged prostate and appropriate treatment prescribed. If the enlargement of the prostate and the urination problems are relatively mild then it is usually left for a period of time to see if the normal reduction in testosterone will result in a decrease in the size of the prostate.

If the enlargement of the prostate or the symptoms warrant medical intervention it is usual to prescribe either alpha-blockers (can have some nasty side effects) or a testosterone lowering drug. As the testosterone levels decrease the prostate shrinks and the urination problems are solved. However there are obvious side effects such as loss of sex drive and possible erectile problems.

Obviously, the more serious disease to consider is prostate cancer and this is why it is vital that men over the age of 50 book themselves in with the doctor at least once a year for a thorough MOT. Men are notorious for putting off going to the doctor with minor symptoms and that is why it is estimated that 18 million men over the last five years have ended up being on medication for life or facing radical surgery because they left it too late for a more simple approach to fixing the problem.

In the second part of the book I introduce you to certain foods that contain nutrients that have traditionally been used to help prevent prostate enlargement and including them in your daily diet will certainly do you no harm. Again I must emphasise that if you are already on medication to reduce an enlarged prostate you should not suddenly stop taking it. Follow the healthy eating plan and after a number of weeks ask your doctor to evaluate your need for the medication.

Summary

- There are a number of factors that affect sexual performance but one of the areas that is often overlooked is the connection to diet and the lack of certain nutrients essential for healthy hormone production.
- Damage to the external reproductive organs such as the testes or the penis can result in ED.
- Certain prescription drugs whilst addressing one problem may create another.
- Young men should be aware of how their lifestyle choices today might impact on their ability to father children in the future or affect their sex lives in middle age.

7. The Endocrine System & Hormones

We cannot look at the male reproductive system and organs without including the endocrine system as well. This is the system that produces not only the sex hormones but also the other hormones necessary for the healthy growth and development of every cell, organ and function within our bodies. Usually responsible for the slower processes such as cell growth the endocrine glands and hormones will also work with other systems such as the nervous system to ensure the smooth running of processes like breathing and movement.

Glands

A gland is a group of cells that produce and secretes chemicals from materials that it has selected from the bloodstream. It processes these raw materials and either secretes the end product in specific areas such as the salivary glands or sweat glands in the case of the exocrine glands or directly back into the bloodstream from the endocrine system.

The main glands that make up the endocrine system are the hypothalamus, pituitary (master gland), thyroid, parathyroids, adrenals, pineal, ovaries and testes. The pancreas is also part of the endocrine system but is associated more with the digestive system and digestive enzymes. Although this book is focussing on the male reproductive system it is important to understand how all our glands and hormones work together to enable the human body to be fit enough to complete the reproductive cycle.

Hormones

Hormones are some of the most powerful chemical messengers found in the body and are secreted by glands that transfer information and instructions from one set of cells to another. They circulate throughout the body but will only affect those cells that have been programmed to respond to their specific message. All hormone levels can be influenced by our general health, stress levels and the balance of fluid and minerals such as salt in the bloodstream. This is the reason that it is necessary to have a healthy and balanced lifestyle and diet to ensure the reproductive system is functioning as it should.

Most of us when we talk about hormones are usually referring to the reproductive ones such as testosterone, progesterone and oestrogen. 'It must be your hormones' is a very common phrase used when we girls are suffering from PMS or sometimes even when we are not, according to whom is talking!

We all know that as we get older our reproductive hormones decrease and both men and women go through a menopause. Women are more affected by this obviously, but men too experience a decrease in testosterone levels and the changes that this brings about including a reduction in sexual performance.

However, our sex hormones are just three of the many hormones that are produced in our bodies and even though our reproductive abilities may decrease as we get older, the hormones involved are still active within our body. If they and our other hormones are looked after they will contribute to a healthy, energetic and youthful appearance. Sex does not stop when we get middle aged and maintaining a good diet and active lifestyle influence a healthy and functioning reproductive system. It should be possible to enjoy our sexuality into our 70's and 80's and achieve just as much pleasure as in our youth. A young man at his peak of sexual performance probably gives little thought to the process but if he concentrated more on what he was putting into his own body at that age he would reap the benefits 30 or 40 years later!

Each gland within the endocrine system may produce one or more different hormone to affect a process in the body. For example the pancreas secretes Insulin, glucagon and Stomostatin. Insulin and glucagon are secreted according to the level of blood sugar and Stomostatin is the referee to ensure that not too much of either is secreted and therefore blood sugar levels remain balanced. If you are suffering from diabetes and on medication then you may well suffer from ED. Whilst it does not sound very sexy, looking after your pancreas does affect your sex life!

Hormones are manufactured from components of food, which means that the type of diet you follow has a major impact on keeping hormone levels in balance. Hormones are either protein-like as in insulin, or fat like as in steroid hormones.

Whatever the level of hormones produced by particular glands, if they are not communicating when they get to their destination such as the thyroid gland, kidneys, testes or ovaries they will not be effective and the ongoing functions they are supposed to stimulate will be under effective. This includes the reproductive process which requires the balance of most of the hormones for successful production, fertilisation and then development of the egg by a sperm and our sexual drive and performance.

Glands & Hormones in the Endocrine System

The Hypothalamus

As I have already said, sexual performance is a mental, physical and emotional response to various stimuli.

Sex starts in the head and you will understand that when you see what the hypothalamus actually controls in the body.

The other name of the hypothalamus is actually the word homeostasis, which means balance, which is very appropriate. It is located in the middle of the base of the brain and is connected to the pituitary lobes, which form the most important gland in the body and is often referred to as the Master Gland.

The hypothalamus regulates body temperature, blood sugar, water balance, fat metabolism, appetite, body weight, sensory input like taste and smell and sight, sleep, sexual behaviour, emotions, hormone productions, menstrual cycle regulation and the automatic nervous system that controls automatic functions such as breathing and the heart muscle.

To put this into perspective and relate it back to the questionnaire at the beginning of the book we are looking at regulating our body's blood pressure, cholesterol, blood sugar levels, hormone production and reproductive system health.

It is often inferred that men only think with their penis when it comes to sex so it should be of some comfort to understand that in fact it is all in your head!

As far as reduced sexual performance is concerned it is the Hypothalamus that will benefit the most from a healthy diet and lifestyle.

The Pituitary Gland

The pituitary gland has an anterior and posterior lobe. The anterior lobe regulates the activity of the thyroid, adrenals and the reproductive glands producing a number of hormones.

- *Growth hormone* stimulates the growth of bone and body tissues and plays a part in the metabolism of nutrients and minerals.
- *Prolactin*, which activates milk production in mothers who are breastfeeding.
- *Thyrotropin* which stimulates the thyroid to produce hormones.
- *Corticotrophin* which stimulates the adrenal glands to produce its hormones.
- *Gonadotrophs* are cells that secret the two hormones that stimulate hormone production in the ovaries and testes. These are called *luteinising hormone* and *follicle stimulating hormone* and whilst not essential to life are essential to reproduction.

The pituitary gland also secretes endorphins, which act as natural pain relief within the nervous system. It is also the gland that releases hormones that signal the ovaries and testes to make the sex hormones and controls the ovulation and menstrual cycle.

The posterior lobe of the pituitary has two main functions one of which is the release of a hormone to control water balance through its affect on the kidneys and urine output. The second is the release of oxytocin the trigger for contractions of the womb during labour.

The Thyroid

It may seem strange to be looking at non sexual glands when talking about sexual dysfunction but you have to take the body as a whole and if one organ, gland or system is not functioning correctly then it will have a knock on affect on the rest of the body. Since factors causing sexual dysfunction include chronic fatigue and depression having a healthy thyroid is essential.

The thyroid is located in the front of the lower neck and is shaped like a bow tie. It produces the hormones thyroxine and triiodothyronine which are responsible for the speed with which cells burn fuel to provide energy. This is our metabolism or the speed at which we operate. The production and release of these two hormones is controlled by Thyrotropin, which is secreted by the pituitary gland.

The thyroid needs iodine and selenium to produce an enzyme, which converts the amino acid tyrosine into thyroxine. If thyroxine is at a less than optimum level there will be weight gain, fatigue, intestinal problems and thickening skin. Also this gland produces a hormone that is responsible for calcium balance between blood and bones. If this is not working then too much calcium is leeched from the bones leaving them vulnerable to osteoporosis.

The Parathyroids
Attached to the thyroid are four tiny glands that release parathyroid hormone that is responsible with calcitonin, also produced in the thyroid, for calcium balance between blood and bones.

The Adrenal Glands
The Adrenal glands are actually situated on top of each kidney and comprise two parts. The first is the cortex, which produces hormones called corticosteroids, which determine male characteristics, sex drive, stress response, metabolism and the excretion of sodium and potassium from the kidneys. If your adrenal glands are not healthy then it is likely that you will have an underactive sex drive and therefore performance.

The second part of the gland is the medulla, which produces catecholamines such as epinephrine (adrenaline) to increase blood pressure and heart rate in times of danger or stress.

If your stress levels remain high for long periods of time there will be an effect on the rest of your body. The body slows down digestion, maintenance and repair so that it is ready to run for its life at any moment. It definitely speeds up the ageing process because like anything that is not maintained it slowly deteriorates. It will have a very big impact on all the rest of the hormones in the body including your sex drive, which is why stress plays a very important role in problems such as erectile dysfunction and infertility.

The Pineal Gland
This gland is located in the middle of the brain and secretes melatonin the hormone that regulates sleep cycles. Being tired all the time will certainly not help maintain a healthy hormone balance nor your sex life.

Ovaries And Testes

Don't forget that this book is aimed at both men and women and it is important to remember the woman's role in a male's sexual dysfunction.

As a woman ages her own sex drive takes a beating as her hormone levels reduce and become imbalanced through the pre-menopausal, menopausal and post menopausal stages. A willing partner is always an advantage particularly when extra time is required by both for arousal. Understanding how your partner might be feeling from a hormone perspective may help you relax and not feel quite so conscious of your own issues.

The ovaries and the testes are known as the gonads and are the main source for the sexual hormones. The ovaries secrete oestrogen and progesterone as needed, particularly in girls who have reached puberty and are developing breasts and layers of fat around the hips and thighs that would be used primarily to nourish a foetus during pregnancy. Both hormones regulate the menstrual cycle, which is why an imbalance can cause irregular periods or infertility.

Oestrogen hormones include estradiol, oestrone and estriol and as well as their role in the developing female they also have important effects on organs outside of the reproductive system. In fact they have an effect on over 300 different tissues throughout a woman's body including in the central nervous system, liver and the urinary tract. One of their functions is in maintaining bone mass as a woman ages, particularly after the menopause. They also have a positive effect on blood fat and therefore help prevent atherosclerosis and possible heart disease. As we age our skin tends to thicken and oestrogen hormones help preserve the elasticity of the skin as well as promote a sense of general well being.

Progesterone has duties also outside of its reproductive remit and that is its influence on body temperature. This is why taking your temperature every morning during the month can help you pinpoint when you might be ovulating.

As these hormones diminish so does the activity within the ovaries. They become smaller and lighter and the blood vessels that supply them atrophy. The follicles decrease in number and fewer and fewer eggs are produced sometimes skipping several months at a time resulting in irregular periods. Eventually egg production ceases completely as does menstruation and after twelve months you are usually unlikely to conceive.

We covered the testes in the last chapter but it is comforting to know that both men and women face the same issues as they age and that again diet and lifestyle affects both equally when it comes to the health of their reproductive organs and systems.

Summary

- Our sex lives are governed by the master glands in our brain that regulate hormone levels and therefore our internal messaging service. The expression "the mind is willing but the body is weak" is quite true. For a healthy and active sex life we need to be firing on all cylinders which means healthy brain and body.
- Although this book is primarily about men's sexual health it is necessary to consider that our partner's hormonal balance needs to be taken into consideration. As we age it might take a little longer to reach arousal due to hormonal changes but that does not mean that it has to be less pleasurable.
- Taking care of the non-sexual glands is very important as they perform essential activities within the body that keep us feeling energetic and also functioning at the healthiest level for our age.
- Fatigue, depression and stress are leading causes of sexual dysfunction – eating a healthy diet full of the nutrients necessary to fuel the entire system will make sure that our sexual lives remain healthy too.

8. The Obesity Link to Sexual Dysfunction

Before I look at some of the diseases that might be contributing to your lack of sexual performance I am going to start with obesity as it is probably the precursor of most of the other medical problems such as heart disease, diabetes, Acidity, Candida Albicans etc. I will then move onto these in more detail but it is important to remember that this is not a medical reference book and if you feel you are exhibiting any of the symptoms I mention please do go to your doctor and get it checked out. We are not just talking your sex life here but also your life.

Having been very obese at one time in my life I fully sympathise with the notion that being fat is not sexy. It is a combination of perceptions about our own body and the perceptions that we project onto our partner. We assume that if we cannot find our bodies sexy then no one else is going to. Forget love and familiarity, if your self esteem is rock bottom then it is difficult enough to raise a smile, let alone anything else.

Having said that, we have already accepted that there is mental and emotional aspects to sexual dysfunction and whilst later in the book I will take a look at some foods that are allegedly aphrodisiacs, I am not a sex therapist and I suggest that if you feel that you need more advice in that area that you find yourself a registered counsellor.

This book is about lifestyle and diet and the key is to get to the fitness level that allows you to enjoy any form of sexual activity you wish.

To that end you need to determine if weight is part of the issue for you and if it is causing some of the contributory factors to ED. For example, being overweight can lead to high blood pressure and medication, elevated cholesterol and medication, diabetes and medication and chronic diseases such as arthritis and medication.

Being in pain does nothing for your sex drive especially chronic joint pain. If both you and your partner are both suffering from a chronic condition such as arthritis then the chances of you both you being in the mood is highly unlikely. Apart from that, any medication that you are on for these various ailments is likely to have side effects that include reduced libido or even ED.

As I mentioned earlier in the book, I have often reduced clients of 20 stone to tears of hysterical laughter when I have informed them that they are suffering from malnutrition. Our perception of malnourishment is a result of harrowing pictures of starving children and their parents who are surviving on virtually no sustenance at all.

The truth is that obese people may be getting more than enough calories and fat but the food that they are consuming is nutritional poor and here is an example of what I mean.

Diet one

- 3 Mars bars
  = *1,500 calories* (approx)

Plus of course lots of fats and sugars.

Diet Two

Bowl of cereal, with fresh fruit and tea.

- Apple and orange
- Chicken salad with tomato, lettuce, cucumber, and some new potatoes
- 2 Ryvita with low fat cream cheese
- Roasted salmon with carrots, broccoli and two tablespoons of brown rice.
- Bowl of fresh fruit salad and yoghurt.
  = *1,500 calories* (approx)

No prizes for guessing which is better for your body!

Every process in your body requires a specific set of nutrients to function efficiently. I would not have known a vitamin or mineral let alone an amino acid if it had stood up and slapped me in the face until I was in my 40's. Frankly, nutrients are not the sexiest topic and are up there somewhere between train spotting and stamp collecting. However, the fuel that our body requires to be healthy and fire on all cylinders is comprised of this complex soup of nutrients and the resulting chemical reactions. Our brains don't function; the Hypothalamus fails to send the correct messages out to the pituitary gland which is responsible for so many of our life giving functions.

White flour products such as bread, white rice and pasta are not nutritious and this is widely recognised by the manufacturing industry who then try and put back the nutrients extracted with artificial supplementation. When you read about whole grains in the second half of the book you will hopefully realise how much the B vitamins example contribute to your obesity problem and your sex life.

At the back of the book you will find some appendices which will give you the main nutrients that you should be including in your diet and why. Eating fresh fruit and vegetables is essential and many of them over the years have been designated as aphrodisiacs in their own right. That you will have to judge for yourselves but there is no doubt that they provide many of the nutrients necessary for healthy hormones as well as the functioning of our reproductive systems.

Dehydration is a very common cause of many system failures within the body and it also contributes to obesity, high blood pressure, fatigue and lack of libido. Drinking coffee and tea does contribute to your daily allowance but drinking too much caffeine can affect your body in a negative way too. Drinking water has become unfashionable unless it comes from extortionately priced bottles of so called 'mineral water'. Not only that, I have worked with clients who suffered from high blood pressure that were adding to the problem by drinking mineral water with very high sodium contents. Take a look at the nutritional data on a bottle of high priced sparkling bottled water next time you are in the supermarket and multiply the sodium content by 2.5% to get that amount of salt you are consuming!

Willpower

Half the problem with losing weight or getting healthy involves getting your head around willpower.

Willpower is not something we are born with and as children we are not expected to exhibit much particularly when it comes to eating or not eating foods we love. The important issue here is to focus on what you are going to gain rather than what you are going to have to give up.

To put things into perspective when looking at your current lifestyle you need to review exactly how you feel on a physical, mental and emotional level. Are you fed up with feeling bloated, overweight, tired, emotional and guilty and having a poor sex life?

One of the most important lessons that I learnt at 42 years old was that it was okay to say 'NO'. When it came to food it was not in my vocabulary and I realised that I said yes all the time to virtually everything so that everybody liked me. I even kept on saying 'YES' to myself despite all the warnings about my health.

My body has adjusted to a different way of eating and anything that is too fatty, salty, sweet or processed makes it react negatively.

You may be saying to yourself that your body does not react at all to the foods that you eat but you cannot see beneath your skin. Most of us don't know there is a problem with our major organs until something fails and we seek medical help. Unfortunately, our clogged arteries are not visible, nor are the fat layers around our heart and kidneys.

Next time you are in the butchers ask them to show you kidneys that still have the fat around them. If you have a high fat diet, particularly with fried foods and hydrogenated fats then you will have large quantities of unhealthy fat around your major organs.

Later in the book you will find some home truths about some of the processed foods that we eat or drink on a daily basis. Hopefully it will make you think twice about putting them in your mouth quite so regularly.

On the subject of eating high fat and high sugar foods regularly, you may be interested in the Fat accumulation table which shows you the accumulated body fat you will gain per year by eating common snack foods on a daily basis.

I often hear clients say *"but I only eat two digestives a day with my tea"*. Those two digestive biscuits per day = 150 calories per day times 365 = 54,750 calories per year or **16 lbs in body fat**.

Combine this with the other high fat, sugar and calories foods you might be snacking on and you may have the reason why you are 3 stone or 42 lbs overweight right there! If you only said "NO" to half the snacks you are currently consuming you would find the process of losing weight much more effective and rapid.

Willpower is about making a decision, making a plan, sticking to it, setting reasonable goals and expectations and rewarding yourself when you achieve them. It also means not beating yourself up when you don't make a target, but rationally changing the game plan so that you achieve it next week. This does not mean diving into a large pizza and tub of ice cream nor should these be considered rewards.

Fat Accumulation Table

FOOD ITEM (PER DAY)	Calories per Portion	Lbs of body fat gained per Year
Apple (4 oz)	40	4
Beef (6 oz)	300	31
Beer per pint (7 units a week)	180	19
Biscuit, average (x 2)	200	20
Biscuit, chocolate (x 2)	180	19
Biscuit, digestive (x 2)	150	16
Bread, wholemeal, 1 slice	90	9
Breakfast, cereal (2 oz)	180	18
Breakfast, Fried sausage, bacon, egg	500	52
Breakfast, Grilled (poached egg)	350	36
Butter (2 oz; eating or cooking)	412	43
Cheese, cheddar, full-fat (3 oz)	345	36
Cheese, cheddar, half-fat (3 oz)	219	23
Chicken (6 oz)	210	22
Chicken Kiev (5 oz)	375	39
Chocolate snack bar (50 g)	260	27
Chocolate bar, Milk (100 g/3.5 oz)	530	56
Cod (baked or grilled; 6 oz)	160	17
Cod in batter (fried; 6 oz)	415	43
Cream crackers (x 4)	140	15
Cream, full-fat (1 oz)	126	13
Cream, single (1 oz)	55	6
Crispbread (x 2)	54	6
Croissant (standard size)	215	22
Danish Pastry (6 oz)	650	68
Doughnut (jam; 3 oz)	250	26
Flapjack	350	36
Frosted nut flakes	260	27

Fat Accumulation Table

FOOD ITEM (PER DAY)	Calories per Portion	Lbs of body fat gained per Year
Fruit cake (3 oz)	300	31
Fruit muffin	400	42
Fruit, dried (4 oz)	350	36
Ham (6 oz)	180	19
Ice cream (luxury mixed; 3 oz)	250	26
Ice cream (vanilla; 3 oz)	150	16
Milk, full-fat (half pint)	220	23
Milk, semi-skimmed (half pint)	180	19
Milk, skimmed (half pint)	93	10
Orange (4 oz)	80	8
Peanuts (roasted; 2 oz)	338	35
Pear (4 oz)	65	7
Pizza, deep-crust (1 a week)	1,100	16
Pizza, thin-crust (1 a week)	750	11
Porridge oats (2 oz)	200	20
Potato crisps (1 oz packet)	150	16
Potato crisps (low-fat; 1 oz)	130	14
Reduced-fat spread (2 oz)	218	23
Salmon (grilled; 6 oz)	360	37
Salsa (1 oz)	11	2
Shortbread (1 oz x 2)	280	30
Sour cream dip (1 oz)	101	11
Tuna, canned, in brine (6 oz)	168	17
Tuna, canned, in oil (6 oz)	312	33
Vegetable protein (6 oz)	144	15
Wine per medium glass	100	10

Notes for the Fat Accumulation Table

- The food items are arranged in alphabetical order
- The table shows some of the common foods that can become a daily or weekly habit with people.
- You may hear people say, for example, that they only have *"two chocolate biscuits a day"* or *"only one pizza"* or *"a few pints a week"*. Not being aware of the calories consumed **cumulatively** in the course of a few months, or a year, can cause extra weight to creep on over a period of time.
- Take a look at the largest numbers in lbs/Kg columns to see the foods that can cause the biggest problems.
- Note too the portion sizes that are used in the table. If your portion size is larger, or smaller, then remember to make the appropriate corrections.
- You will note that I have included Salmon which I consider to be a food essential in everyone's diet. However, even superfoods like this can contribute to weight gain if used every day. Salmon as a healthy fatty fish should be included two or three times a week as should non-salty nuts such as walnuts. If the rest of your diet is made up of unprocessed, natural vegetables, fruits and grains eating foods such as salmon is great.

For example

- The portion size for Vanilla Ice Cream is shown as 3 oz (85 grams) and this has annual penalty of 16 lbs a year.
- However, if you are in the habit of having half a pint of ice cream as the portion (around 7½ oz) the penalty suddenly goes up to 39 lbs per annum!

Research Notes:

On the subject of Salmon, a recent study, published in 2013 by the Queen Mary University of London, found that eating Salmon twice a week could protect against skin cancer.

Omega-3 fatty acids found in oily fish, which includes sardines, mackeral and trout, destroy malignant cells in skin and mouth tumours. Experiments also found that the omega-3 fatty acids induced cell death in both early and later stages of the disease.

9. Getting to a Healthier Weight

It is important to have a start point when you are planning to lose weight so that you have a road map, with a destination that you can follow. I often hear clients say 'I would just love to lose 10 kilos or 2 stone or 10 lbs'. This is based not necessarily on the actual weight they need to lose but an acceptably achievable goal. To be honest you need to be a little more specific than this. You may only need to lose 7 lbs or 5 kilos or you may need to lose more to reach a healthy weight for your age and activity level.

In the last part of the book you will find a healthy eating plan that can be adjusted for your current weight and fitness level but in this section I want to give you a couple of tools to use to determine what your healthy weight should be.

There are two common methods of measuring your weight with regard to health and that is a straightforward weight/height/ sex comparison and BMI or Body Mass Index. I will look at them both but I believe that it is easier to manage and track your actual weight rather than BMI.

Most ideal weight profiles are derived from an insurance company ideal weight table. This however was produced in 1959 when physically we were shorter and our diet following the war years was still restricted for many people. I don't believe that this table is appropriate today and if you take the ideal weights in that table and treat it as the minimum weight for your height then I believe that it is more realistic for this generation.

It is a guideline only and the important factors are the indicators of how healthy you are internally as well as externally. Of greater importance to me, are your blood pressure, cholesterol and blood sugar levels. Are you exercising regularly and have plenty of energy and for the purposes of this book, are you enjoying a great sex life?

Working Out What You Should Weigh

For medium framed women; as a base use 100 lbs up to five feet and then add 6 lbs for every inch over that height. Modify by 5% either way if you have a light frame or heavy frame.

For example: a woman who has a heavy frame and is 5' 6" would have an optimal weight of 100 lbs + 36 lbs = 136 lbs x 5% = 6.8 lbs giving an optimum weight of 136.8 lbs (or 62.2 Kilos.)

For medium framed men; as a base use 106 lbs up to five feet and then add 7 lbs for every inch over that height. Modify by 5% either way if you have a light frame or heavy frame.

For example: a light framed man of 5' 6" would be 106 lbs + 70 lbs = 176 lbs less 5% = 9 lbs = 167 lbs (or 75.9 Kilos.)

This is not exact, but it gives you an approximate idea of where you should be. To be honest I have met people who are fantastically healthy, fit and full of energy who are a stone or even two stone heavier. But there is no doubt that – if we are talking about being full of life and sex appeal – being a healthy weight for your age and size is important.

Body Mass Index

What Is Body Mass Index?

This is a statistical measurement which was invented in the mid 1800's by a Belgian Adolphe Quetelet as a social statistic for the general population, not as a measurement for individuals.

The formula used today takes the individual's body weight divided by the square of their height. What it does not take into consideration is the muscle mass of the individual, for example an athlete or body builder may have a very high BMI but be very fit.

I use it as a guideline only as I prefer to look at a number of factors which I have already mentioned which include healthy weight for age and sex of the individual coupled with normal key indicators of blood pressure, cholesterol and blood sugar.

If you wish to work out your BMI here is the formula and what the resulting figure might mean. Use it by all means in combination with the other measurements.

Certainly if you are not a professional athlete or bodybuilder the higher the BMI the greater the risk of you developing health problems such as heart disease, diabetes and cancer which will be contributory factors to sexual dysfunction.

Your BMI Is Calculated Using This Formula:

$$BMI = (Weight) \div (Height)^2$$

Where Weight is in kg and height is in metres

A BMI of below 16.5 is considered to be starvation and is unfortunately becoming quite common in teenage girls who are suffering from eating disorders such as Anorexia.

BMI of below 18 may indicate that you are underweight but again if you look at marathon runners who are very slight and muscular this is not always true and these factors need to be taken into account such as your daily calorie intake.

BMI of between 19 and 24 is considered to be the healthy range and people within this band less likely to be at risk of developing obesity related health problems.

BMI of between 25 and 29 is considered to indicate that the individual is overweight but as in previous bands other factors such as muscle mass need to be taken into account. If you are within this band you are put at a moderate risk of developing risk factors for your health.

BMI of 30 and over is considered to indicate obesity and therefore the band that indicates the highest risk of developing weight related health issues. Again other factors need to be taken into consideration. If you are not an athlete or bodybuilder then you need to use this measurement in conjunction with your weight and work to reduce both to healthier levels.

It is important not to just use one measurement in isolation. I prefer to use weight and key health indicators such as BP, Cholesterol and Blood Sugar in combination.

Remember that being very overweight will put enormous stress on all the operating systems in your body and as such you will be running substantially under par in all areas of your health including your sex life.

If it is any consolation to those of you who are not looking forward to the reduced calorie eating programme you will find that you will be eating six times a day and all the food is delicious and nutrient packed and you should never be hungry.

Exercise

If you are a couch potato you are affecting the health of your body and your ability to function on many levels including in your sex life.

We were born to move and if you don't then you will become prone to problems such as high blood pressure, heart disease, obesity, lack of energy, poor muscle tone, bone disease and chronic problems such as arthritis.

I am not as slim as I would like to be but that is a fashion statement rather than a health issue. I walk every day and also include separate walks at a more aerobic level, but importantly the key indicators that I mentioned earlier including blood pressure, cholesterol and blood sugar are all in normal range.

If you have not been exercising at all then don't throw yourself out the door and run for five miles as you will do more harm than good.

At the back of the book you will find a programme that will ease you into walking first and then some ideas for other forms of exercise that will benefit rather than harm you. One of the sexiest forms of exercise is Yoga which will certainly improve both your muscle tone and your flexibility. If you feel that you cannot face a group class then there are some excellent DVDs available that you can work with at home. To get you started and to help you ease into a more strenuous exercise programme you will find breathing and flexibility exercises that will have an impact on not only your health but your sex life too.

I will be covering many of these topics in more detail at the back of the book and in the meantime we need to look at the other contributory factors that affect your sex drive and performance.

Summary

- When we look in the mirror and we are overweight this will often affect how we feel about ourselves sexually. We project these emotions onto our partners and this leads to both inhibition and loss of sex drive.
- Very obese men and women are often suffering from malnutrition – they get plenty of fat and calories but only in foods that are usually full of processed rubbish too. Their bodies are deprived of all the natural ingredients necessary not only to be a healthy weight but also to manufacture the hormones necessary to fuel our libido.

- Willpower is a matter of putting a different set of priorities first. Do you want a great, energetic and fit body with a healthy erection or do you really want to eat another chocolate biscuit?
- We should not stigmatise obesity but we should also recognise that we are responsible for what we put in our mouths so next time you are naked in front of the mirror celebrate your curves but make your mind up to get rid of the bulges.
- You need a plan and that plan begins when you admit what your real weight is!
- Get on the scales – then use the simple calculation from earlier in the chapter to decide what weight you should be.
- Use the healthy eating plan at the back of the book to get you started and then sit down and work out an exercise programme that eases you into getting your body fitter.

10. Lifeblood

One of the constituents of our bodies that we tend to take for granted is our blood. Women have a closer connection with blood on a regular basis, during menstruation, and we have all cut ourselves and slapped a plaster over the damage and not thought much of it. However, blood is alive with an incredibly complex group of components completing several vital roles every second of every day to ensure that we stay alive. As well as giving us life it should also enable all of our organs to perform efficiently and this includes our sexual organs that rely heavily on blood flow for arousal.

If our blood is not healthy we can suffer from anaemia, inefficient immune systems, slow healing and frequent infections. Long term blood disorders lead to much more serious illnesses such as cancer and organ failure.

Without a microscope we are unable to see the amazing life that is contained in just one small drop of blood which makes it easy to take it for granted. Once you understand some of the properties and duties of your blood, it will be easy to make sure that you include foods in your diet that promote its health and therefore your own.

The Cardiovascular System

In Chapter Eleven I will focus on the cardiovascular system's function, to pump our blood around the body. If this process stops for more than a few seconds we will lose consciousness. Every part of our body requires oxygen and nutrients on demand, including additional supplies when we are under pressure. Our cardiovascular system deals with this process without any thought or involvement from us and in addition it will remove any waste products from our systems at the same time. A healthy cardiovascular system is essential and the quality of our blood is vital to our survival.

Blood is a liquid tissue and your body contains around twelve pints, without which you would die. It performs a number of crucial functions within the body, including the transportation of oxygen and carbon dioxide, food molecules (glucose, fats and amino acids), ions, waste (such as urea), hormones and heat around the body. One of its major functions is the defence of the body against infections and other ingested toxins.

The Components of Blood and the Immune System

Within blood is plasma, which is the pale yellow liquid that can easily be replaced by your body when it needs to. It is mainly water and proteins which assist your body in controlling bleeding and fighting infection. It is essential for the circulation of our red and white blood cells and platelets and also ensures that our natural, chemical communication system is operational. This communication system reaches every part of the body via the capillaries and is fuelled by minerals, vitamins, hormones and antibodies.

What Are the Different Blood Cell Types?

- **Red blood cells, or erythrocytes,** are the most numerous type of blood cell. They are shaped specifically to ensure that they absorb as much oxygen from the lungs as possible. In just one minute 120 million of your red blood cells will die but in the same time frame exactly the same amount will be replaced from the bone marrow. The process actually starts in the kidneys, which release a hormone called erythropoietin, which travels to the bone marrow where it stimulates the production of erythrocytes. This is another reason why it is so vital to maintain the function of your kidneys with a diet rich in nutrients.
- **White blood cells** are called leukocytes and there are five types carrying out specific roles within the blood. **Neutrophils, Eosinophils, Lymphocytes, Monocytes** and **Basophils**.
- **Neutrophils** are the most abundant of the white blood cells and are the first line of defence. They squeeze through the capillaries to infected areas in the body and consume and destroy invading bacteria and viruses. Even when we are healthy this process is essential as we are constantly ingesting, absorbing or inhaling harmful substances in our everyday environment. If our blood is healthy and well populated with Neutrophils we can prevent these invasions leading to illness and disease.

- **Eosinophils** are not very abundant in the blood but they are on stand-by and can increase their numbers dramatically if the body comes under attack from certain types of parasites. The cell will rush to the infected area such as the intestines and release a toxic substance over the parasite to destroy it.
- **Lymphocytes** are the name given to a group of different cells with a specific role within the immune system.
- **B-Lymphocytes** (B Cells) are responsible for making our antibodies in response to an infection.
- **T-Lymphocytes** (T-Cells) are a family of cells including Inflammatory T-cells that rally Neutrophils and macrophages to the site of an infection quickly where they will consume bacteria.
- **Cytotoxic T-Lymphocytes** that kill virus infected and possibly cancerous tumour cells.
- **Helper T-Cells** that enhance the production of antibodies.
- **Monocytes** leave the blood and become **macrophages**, which are large cells that ingest and destroy any invading antigens that enter the body and also any dead and dying cells from the body.
- **Basophils** also increase production during an infection and will leave the bloodstream via the capillaries and collect at the site of an infection where they will discharge granules that will stimulate the release of histamine, serotonin, prostaglandins and **leukotrines**. This increases the flow of blood to the infected site and results in an inflammatory reaction. An example of this might be a wasp sting or an allergic reaction to ingesting pollen resulting in a hay-fever attack.

What Else Is in the Blood That Is So Vital for Our Health?

We have already established that without blood we die and we need a system in place that ensures that any break in the circulatory system is plugged and repaired as quickly as possible.

- **Platelets** are fragments of cells and must be kept at sufficient density in the blood to ensure that when blood vessels are cut or damaged the loss of blood can be stopped before shock and possible death occurs. This is accomplished by a process called coagulation or clotting.

A clot is formed when platelets form a plug, which is enmeshed in a network of insoluble fibrin molecules. This forms over any break in the circulatory system preventing any further loss of blood.

Other Functions of the Blood

We have an absolute necessity for oxygen to ensure our survival. It is unlikely that you will survive longer than six minutes without breathing in oxygen, but it is also vitally important for the survival of every cell within the body. If an area of the cardiovascular system is damaged and oxygen is unable to reach the tissues directly affected then that tissue will die and the infection generated will compromise the health of the rest of the body. The most vulnerable parts of the body are the hands and feet where irreparable damage to the tiny network of capillaries could lead to amputation.

The red blood cells are responsible for the transportation of both oxygen and carbon dioxide within the haemoglobin in the blood.

As important as breathing in and utilising oxygen is concerned, getting rid of the carbon dioxide waste, which is produced during this process, is equally important. Some carbon dioxide produced in the tissues is processed and converted to a harmless substance that can be eliminated easily but some has to be transported via the bloodstream back to the lungs to be got rid of.

Other Transportation Duties

Substances in the bloodstream like cholesterol and other fats are transported around the body, from originating organs like the liver, to elimination points where they are removed from the blood and either absorbed into cells or processing points such as the kidneys. This process is used to transport glucose and sugars, hormones and waste products like urea that becomes urine.
We are an extremely efficient waste producer and it is when this waste is not eliminated safely, and regularly, from the body that we become ill and diseased.

One of the causes of sexual disinterest let alone dysfunction is tiredness. Not the everyday, working hard, physical labour or activity kind of tiredness but bone weariness. This can be a result of insufficient nutrients within your diet causing mild to serious anaemia. This can go undetected for a long time so it is important to recognise when your tiredness and lack of libido might be down to something a little more serious. It is a simple test and is important not to put off.

Anaemia

There are actually several types of Anaemia but I am just going to focus on two that will give you an idea of how important our blood health is. *Iron deficiency Anaemia* and *Pernicious Anaemia* sometimes also known as Megoblastic Anaemia. This anaemia is a Vitamin Deficiency anaemia and so both are preventable in most cases and can be treated with diet.

Iron deficiency Anaemia is one of the most common types and is usually associated with women. Mostly in pregnancy, but it can also affect women who have suffered heavy periods throughout their reproductive lives. As the name implies, it is caused by the lack of iron.

There are also other causes of blood loss, such as surgery or internal bleeding, but there are some diseases such as chronic bowel problems that induce a slow loss of blood over a long period of time and this can lead to Anaemia.

Later in the book I will take a closer look at Candida Albicans, a parasite that robs nutrients from your food for its own use. This means iron too. As a result, part of the chronic fatigue associated with Candida can be linked to mild forms of anaemia.

Of the two anaemias this one is wholly preventable and treatable with changes in diet and in some cases, supplementation.

The key to the diet is not just taking in iron in extra quantities and in fact it is not a good idea to suddenly rush off and grab yourself a bottle of iron tablets and start taking a handful. It is far better to start with adjusting your diet to include foods that are a good source of the mineral.

What Is Pernicious Anaemia?

Pernicious Anaemia is actually a *Vitamin Deficiency* rather than an *iron deficiency*. As well as iron, your body needs B6, B12 and folic Acid, or Folate, to produce enough healthy red blood cells. If your diet is lacking in these, then you will have fewer red blood cells, and therefore less iron, and be anaemic. I will cover the role of Vitamin B6 and the other B vitamins in the nutritional section in the book.

Who Is the Most Likely to Suffer from This Type of Anaemia?

Both men and women suffer from this type of anaemia. In rare cases it can be genetic or congenital when someone is born with the inability to absorb Vitamin B12 from their diet. In this case although a healthy diet will support the sufferer they have to be treated with injections of B12, in some cases for the rest of their lives.

As you will see from the sections on iron and B6, diet plays an enormous part in the prevention and treatment of blood diseases. Today's diet of processed foods, additives, chemicals and fad weight-loss plans are all contributing to the inability of our body to process the necessary and vital nutrients efficiently. I have worked with many people who decide that they are going to become vegetarian and have done so without finding appropriate substitutes for animal products that previously provided nutrients such as iron and the B vitamins. If you wish to become vegetarian then make sure that you are getting sufficient wholegrains, fermented soy products like miso or Tempeh and plenty of fresh fruit and green vegetables.

In some anaemic patients it is the result of a disease or condition that prevents absorption of nutrients in general – such as Candida – Crohns disease or if someone is celiac. Anything that affects the small intestine will cause mal absorption of nutrients and result in possible anaemia

Also, long-term medication, use of the pill, HRT and chemotherapy can have an affect on the way we absorb iron, B6, B12 and Folate. In the case of chemotherapy too many red cells may have been killed and not yet been replaced. As we said earlier, blood-loss means that the iron that is normally recycled when cells die off naturally is not available. It is important that anyone who has been through as intensive a treatment as this make sure that their diet is absolutely optimum for rebuilding this system in their bodies.

What Symptoms Would Someone Experience If They Were Anaemic?

People will vary with the symptoms depending on the severity of the problem.

- Generally people will begin to feel very tired. As we have said the body is being deprived of one of its main energy sources – oxygen.
- Some may experience rapid heartbeats – perhaps find themselves getting breathless when they have not really over exerted themselves.

- There might be some chest pain associated with the symptoms – headaches or dizziness.
- Hands and feet can become numb and very cold.
- Nausea, causing loss of appetite and weight loss.
- Bleeding gums and a yellowish tinge to the skin and around the eyes.

What Should You Do If You Feel That You Might Be Anaemic?

If anyone is suffering from any of the symptoms above and is worried they should go and see their doctor and ask them to do a blood test. It would certainly either put their mind at rest or establish that there is a problem which can be easily treated – if necessary with a short term course of iron supplements or, if the problem is more serious, with injections. For the dietary based anaemias or where it is only a temporary problem with absorption of B12 – diet and supplementation would be used.

If the problem is a long term issue, as with pernicious anaemia, then the treatment usually consists of injections – daily to begin with, for a week or so, until the condition as stabilised and then as required, which might be monthly or three-monthly.

It can be supported by a healthy diet because the body in general will become healthier by absorbing the nutrients that it is able to.

What About Our Diet?

As a preventative and to help the body recover there are certain foods that should be eaten on a regular basis to ensure that we are taking in sufficient iron- B12 – Folate or folic acid, manganese and B6. In the nutritional section of the book you will find which foods are rich in these vitamins and minerals and they are incorporated into the Healthy Eating Plan.

What About Alcohol and Anaemia?

We all know that excessive alcohol consumption is not good for us. As with everything that we have covered on healthy eating – moderation is the key. Alcohol does inhibit the absorption of not only iron but also other essential nutrients such as B6.

However, having said that, stress also plays a part in the way our body processes nutrients. You may find that a glass of red wine every night with your dinner, or if you are out, as part of a healthy eating plan is quite acceptable. We have talked about the benefits of the occasional glass of wine and life is too short to give up everything.

What About Taking Supplements?

If you think that you might be suffering from Anaemia then go to your doctor – be tested and he will evaluate the level of deficiency you are suffering from and the specific amount of either iron, B6 or B12 you might require.

If you are following the healthy eating programme you should be obtaining good levels of the vitamins and minerals. But in times of stress, or as we get older, our ability to digest and absorb nutrients is compromised and we do need some help. I believe in taking a high quality multi-Vitamin and mineral to supplement a healthy eating programme. However, do consult your doctor first and establish if any further supplementation is needed to resolve any issues you might have.

One final note: Iron tablets can make you constipated. I prefer liquid supplements and it is a good idea to ask a pharmacist for one that is kind to your stomach.

Summary

- Blood is absolutely essential to your life and also to the functions within your body.
- Tiredness resulting from mild anaemia could be affecting your sex life so check it out.
- There can be some underlying causes for feeling tired that are not related to anaemia such as Candida Albicans, a mild ongoing infection or lack of nutrients in general.
- Building your immune system can take a little time but following the healthy eating plan with its nutrients for blood health will make a difference.

11. The Circulatory System and High Blood Pressure

As I have already stated earlier in the book, it is important that you understand how the body works to enable you to keep it healthy. Unless we cut ourselves, our blood flow is yet another automatic bodily function that we take for granted. It is also hidden from view and in many cases it is only when there is a system failure that we know something is wrong. If you are unable to achieve or maintain an erection it may well be indicative that it is a wider spread problem that needs to be addressed as quickly as possible. Certainly I advise you to consult your doctor and ask for a check up especially if you have not had your blood pressure, cholesterol and blood sugar checked recently.

There are two circulatory systems working in the body, the pulmonary and the systemic. Apart from major veins and arteries there are millions of smaller blood vessels that form an interconnecting pathway throughout the body. As every man knows it is the blood flow to the penis that affects both the strengths and longevity of an erection. The health of blood vessels is very dependent on your lifestyle choices and if you are starving your body of nutrients and smoke then you can expect to have problems with erections as you age.

How the Circulatory Systems Work

In the pulmonary system deoxygenated blood is taken from the heart to the lungs where it is replenished with oxygen before making the return journey back to the heart. The oxygenated blood leaves the heart in the systemic circulatory network and taken to every single part of the body.

Although the circulation in our bodies is a closed system the blood in the circuit begins its journey around the body in the left ventricle of the heart into the aorta. The blood at this point is oxygen rich and full of nutrients and hormones as well as other substances necessary for us to function.

The coronary arteries split off and the aorta passes upward before doubling back on itself in an arch. From this arch the two main arteries to the head split off (left and right carotid arteries) and the main arteries for the arms (brachial). The aorta descends down the chest and into the abdomen where it branches off to the liver, intestines, and each kidney before dividing into the left and right iliac arteries, which supply blood to the pelvis and the legs. From there the blood passes into the arterioles and capillaries to feed the interior of organs and outlying areas of the body and remove any waste.

After passing through these tiny blood vessels the blood is passed into the veins starting its return journey in small vessels called venules which are similar in size to the arterioles. It then makes it way back to the heart via the veins, which are close to the skin and visible at most times to the naked eye. These are the veins that contain valves to ensure the blood travels in only one direction.

All the veins in the body eventually merge into two very large blood vessels called the superior vena cava and the inferior vena cava. The first collects the blood from the head, arms and neck and the second the blood from the lower half of the body. This blood then passes back into the heart and out to the lungs where it is re-oxygenated and returned to the heart to begin the process all over again.

What Is the Structure of the Different Blood Vessels?

Arteries are subjected to enormous pressure with each strong heartbeat and they therefore have to be thick walled and muscular. The outer layer of the artery (tunica adventitia) is a loose fibrous sheath filled with tiny blood vessels that supply nutrients to the artery walls. Beneath this is an elastic sheath covering the muscular layer (tunica media) that gives the artery its strength. There is an internal elastic area covering the lining (tunica intima) of the blood vessel.

The thick elastic and muscular walls are vital if the system is to work efficiently and the blood is to be pushed around the entire body.

When you take your own pulse you will be measuring the force of each heartbeat as it is transmitted through the arteries and it is a very useful diagnostic tool for a doctor when determining any heart or circulatory problems you might be experiencing.

Veins are similar to arteries in the way that they circulate and when they both service major organs they often run in parallel. The major differences in the two blood vessels are structural to enable them to perform their own individual roles in the circulatory system.

Veins have much thinner and more flexible walls that can expand to hold large volumes of blood. Pressure of blood returning to the heart is much lower than that in the arteries and its movement requires the use of valves in the veins to prevent the blood going backwards in the system.

Capillaries only measure about 8 thousandths of a millimetre and are barely wider than a single blood cell. These minute vessels are thin and porous allowing the nutrients, oxygen rich blood and waste to pass between the circulatory system and the cells freely.

Capillaries also have another vital role in the body and this is in their ability to help regulate our body temperature. When the body is hot the capillaries in the skin expand to allow more blood to reach the surface of the skin and be cooled. When we experience extreme cold our circulatory system closest to the skin will begin to shut down forcing our blood to the centre of our bodies to ensure that our hearts and lungs are protected.

The capillaries nearest the skin are the most vulnerable to cuts and when we bruise it is the damage to these small blood vessels just under the skin which cause the discolouration. During our lifetime any damage is usually repaired but as we age this ability lessens and capillaries collapse and leave the purple patches behind that are commonly seen on the arms and legs of the very elderly.

After passing through the capillaries and having completed the job of providing oxygen and nutrients from the tips of our toes to the scalp tissues the blood returns to the heart in the veins.

Are There Any Interruptions to the Smooth Flow of Blood in Our System?

At some stage food that we have consumed must be processed and the nutrients extracted and waste removed. Part of this process involves the intestines and the liver. When blood leaves the intestines it does not flow directly back to the heart but diverts into the liver or hepatic portal system of veins. Once in the liver this enriched blood passes through the liver cells in special capillaries called sinusoids before passing back into the veins which transport it to the inferior vena cava and then to the heart.

What If We Suffer Damage To One System or Another?

As blood loss and loss of circulation to a part of the body can be fatal, we do have an emergency diversion system that takes over in some areas. In the arms and the legs for example, damage to one artery stimulates another in the same branch to widen to allow more blood to pass through it, maintaining circulation.

During the fight or flight response when adrenaline has been released, during intense activity or after eating, other mechanisms come into play. If you suddenly become more active, blood vessels in the leg will increase in size and those in the intestine shut down so that you get the power where you need it. When you eat a meal the reverse process occurs with blood being directed to the intestines. This is why it is advisable not to exercise too soon after eating a large meal as you will interrupt this major part of the digestive process. This also applies if you are planning to indulge in very active sex straight after a large meal. Your digestive system and sexual organs will be competing for blood and sometimes the intestines win!

Is Blood in Equal Amounts in the Two Systems?

The blood is not evenly distributed in the two systems. If you were to take a snapshot of the circulatory system you would find approximately 12% to 15% in the arteries and veins in and out of the lungs. About 60% will be in the veins and 15% in the arteries with 5% in the capillaries and 10% in the heart. It will also be travelling at different speeds in the various parts of the system leaving the heart quickly at around 30 cm per second and slowing down considerably in the capillary system. It speeds up again in the veins until it reaches the heart travelling around 20 cm per second.

Where Is Our Circulation Controlled From?

When we take a look at the brain you will see that a number of the systems are governed by certain parts of the brain such as hypothalamus. In the case of our circulation there is a small area in the lower part of the brain which is in charge called the vasomotor centre. The vasomotor centre receives messages from the pressure sensitive nerves in the aorta and carotid arteries and if necessary the centre sends out messages to the arterioles that will expand or constrict to control and maintain correct levels. Again clients are often surprised when I emphasise that their sex lives would be better if they took care of their brains more but I think that you can see that if you want the signals of sexual arousal to be responded to with adequate blood flow then you need to pamper the hypothalamus.

Having a healthy circulatory system is vital if we are to enjoy our old age as it is usually the weakness in our blood vessel walls that will let us down in the end. We are going to focus on blood pressure now but we need to also look at cholesterol as well as clogged arteries also restricts blood flow to the various parts of the body including the penis.

What Is Blood Pressure? If you are in your 40's and 50's then I strongly suggest that you get your blood pressure checked at least every three months. Blood pressure cuffs for both arm and wrist are readily available to buy online or in pharmacies and are a vital investment. Get into the habit of taking your blood pressure a couple of times per month. Once in the morning before you get up to check your resting pressure and then again after being moderately active. It is important that your heartbeat and pressure return to normal readings within a few minutes. High blood pressure is becoming increasingly common in both men and women in the 40 – 60 age group and the worrying trend is that once put on medication for blood pressure patients are rarely taken off their prescription. High blood pressure on its own is a contributory factor to ED and so is the medication that is prescribed for it so you have a double whammy.

How It Works

Blood pressure is the measure of the force of the blood pushing against the walls of the arteries. The pressure is measured in units called mm Hg (millimetres of mercury). Your blood pressure is measured by correlating it to the contractions of the heart. When the heart contracts it is called systolic pressure and when the heart is relaxed it is known as diastolic pressure.

The measurement will vary considerably throughout the day being at its lowest when you are at rest and highest after you have been active for a period of time. Standing, sitting and lying down can alter the reading as can emotional stress, pregnancy, smoking and taking prescribed medication.

If you have a blood pressure around the 120/80 mark then it is considered normal. If you are above 140/90 it is considered to be high blood pressure. There are certain conditions where it is important to keep the blood pressure lower than this such as with diabetics or people with kidney disease, whose blood pressure should be below 130/80. Usually a doctor will take your blood pressure over a period of time to determine if it is continuously high or just elevated for a specific reason before prescribing medication.

When your blood pressure is high it means that the heart and the blood vessels are working too hard and if left untreated it can lead to heart attacks and strokes. This is particularly the case if blood pressure measures more than 160/95 all the time.

How Is Blood Pressure Measured?

Blood pressure is usually measured using a blood pressure cuff (sphygmomanometer). You would normally sit quietly for a few minutes beforehand and it is helpful if you have avoided eating, smoking, drinking tea or coffee or being extremely active for about an hour before the measurement is taken. Other variables that may affect the reading are certain medications, nicotine substitutes or caffeine over the counter medications such as cold remedies and you should tell your doctor or nurse that you are taking these.

How Often Should You Have Your Blood Pressure Measured?

A guideline would be that anyone over 20 should get their blood pressure checked every two years. Anyone over 30 years old every 12 months and anyone over 40 should get it checked every 6 months, although I believe that monthly at home will give you a good base line to determine if you have a problem at some stage.

If it is high then it might indicate other problems such as elevated cholesterol levels and you should consult a doctor if he or she is not the person who has taken the reading.

Since children as young as 10 are showing signs of blocked arteries the earlier that this is picked up the better for overall health in later years.

What Sort of Symptoms Might Indicate That You Are Suffering From Elevated Blood Pressure?

If you are suffering from more than one of these symptoms then do go straight to your doctor of if you prefer to a pharmacy where they have the testing machines and get your blood pressure measured immediately.

- Fatigue – not after normal activity but all the time.
- Vision changes or general eye problems.
- Excessive sweating – in a cool room or after minor exertion.
- Nosebleeds.
- Very pale skin or very red skin.
- Palpitations – where you feel that your heart is pounding in your chest – panic attacks.
- Ringing or buzzing in your ears (tinnitus is a circulatory problem)
- Headaches and dizziness.
- Problems achieving or maintaining an erection

Also, keep an eye on how quickly you lose your temper. Do you become more critical and upset with other people more frequently? You might also suddenly become more prone to emotional outbursts. This is about getting to know your body and understanding that everything is connected. None of the organs or major functions of the body work in isolation. There is a knock on effect throughout your entire body when one part is out of kilter. If you listen to your body closely you will notice when things seem different. Being aware of differences in the early stages makes improving the problem with diet and lifestyle changes much more practical and less reliant on medical intervention.

Traditionally men have been at risk at around 55 years old with women being affected later but this is changing. One of the preconditions for elevated blood pressure is hormonal which is why in pregnancy it is very important that blood pressure is managed carefully.

This also applies in the years before and during menopause when a woman's hormonal makeup is changing and can lead to blood pressure changes. I have worked with many women who have been prescribed blood pressure medication during the lead up to and during the menopause who are still taking pills ten years later. This is very worrying because it is likely that the blood pressure will return to normal after the menopause unless there is arterial damage or other underlying causes such as cholesterol. If you have a healthy lifestyle and your cholesterol is normal without the benefit of statins then talk to your doctor about slowly reducing your dosage over a period of time to see if you can stop taking it altogether.

Does Elevated Blood Pressure Need To Be Treated With Medication?

In many cases, if the problem is diagnosed early enough, some simple lifestyle enhancements may be all that is needed and if possible, this should be the first phase of treatment. This requires that you work with your doctor so that he can monitor your progress over a reasonable period of time. Hopefully medication would be the last resort rather than the first.

It is important that you do take action though because, untreated, high blood pressure not only puts a great strain on the blood vessels and the heart, but also seriously impacts our other major organs that depend on unrestricted blood flow such as the liver, brain, kidneys and lungs.

It is also definitely going to affect your sexual performance and if you go back to the list of symptoms you will see that all of them are hardly conducive to a satisfying and enjoyable sex life.

Most people, once they reach their 50's and 60's and who are not athletic and active, will start to suffer from atherosclerosis which is a hardening of the arteries. When you have something that is as rhythmic as blood flow, it needs a flexible tube to carry it. If the lining of the arteries has stiffened and the vessel has lost its flexibility it will be more difficult for the blood to be forced around the body – and the pressure increases.

Can Making Lifestyle Changes Really Affect Blood Pressure Levels?

I have worked with clients from all age groups and I was always amazed by the improvements that even men and women in their 70's, 80's and even 90's could achieve by making changes to their lifestyles.

Our bodies as they age tend to slow down and this includes the digestive process. Nutrients are not as easily absorbed and therefore body functions are affected including sexual performance. The irony is that is that as we age our appetite tends to decrease as well which means that not only are we not eating sufficient food to supply nutrients but our bodies process it inefficiently.

If you look at active 80 and 90 year olds with all their marbles you will usually find that because they are still out there walking, dancing and looking after themselves that they still have a healthy appetite.

Here is a brief look at some of the foods that can help balance cholesterol, provide you with antioxidants to prevent oxidative damage to the LDL (lousy cholesterol) and help keep your blood vessels clear and your blood pressure normal.

I will go into more detail about these foods in the section on 'superfoods' in another section of the book but all of them will contribute to keeping your blood vessels healthy and unblocked and reduce your risk of developing elevated blood pressure levels.

- **Oranges** with their fibre.
- **Oats** with their fibre called beta-glucan which helps lower cholesterol and prevents plaque from forming in your arteries.
- **Green tea** with its antioxidant, which inhibits the enzymes that produce free radicals in the lining of the arteries. This not only prevents plaque from forming but also improves the ratio of LDL (lousy cholesterol) to HDL (healthy cholesterol)
- **Banana** has fibre too, which helps clear the system of debris and keeps the arteries clean.
- **Brown rice** helps keep your cholesterol down and your arteries healthy with its fibre.
- **Walnuts** with monounsaturated fat help lower lipoprotein in the blood. Lipoprotein if you remember causes platelets to clot which in turn can lead to strokes or a cerebral aneurysm. Walnuts also contain B6, which is very important for a healthy cardiovascular system in general.
- **Salmon** with its omega 3 and B6 has the same effect as walnuts.
- All the **vegetables** on the Superfood list are rich in antioxidants, which remove free radicals from the system and also promote the growth of healthy cells and tissue.

- **Onions** in particular, which contain sulphur compounds that along with B6 and chromium help lower homocysteine levels in the blood. Homocysteine causes platelets to clump so that they can attach themselves to the walls of the arteries and block them – one of the major causes of high blood pressure.

What About Exercise and Blood Pressure?

Aerobic activity such as fast walking will stimulate every part of your body but will also encourage blood flow throughout the circulatory system. As I have already mentioned, no programme to improve blood pressure should exclude exercise but you must begin slowly and work your way up to a daily intensive workout.

Later in the book I will take you through a fitness programme that gradually increases your walking activities to a level where you might even consider jogging or running.

Is There One Major Lifestyle Change That You Can Make That Will Make a Substantial Difference To Your Blood Pressure?

There is actually one very lifesaving change that everyone can make to lower their current blood pressure and to prevent a problem in the future. THAT IS …

REDUCE YOUR SALT INTAKE!

So many times I have worked with clients who tell me that they LOVE salt and that they cannot possibly eat any food without it and please don't make them give it up.

Firstly – you do not LOVE salt. You love your parents, your partner, your children, dog, cat and your hamster. You do not LOVE an inanimate object especially one that has the ability to kill you. Your daily recommended salt intake is one level teaspoon and that includes all food you cook for yourself and in any processed food you consume. You need to multiply any sodium included in food labels by 2.5 to establish exactly how much salt there is a portion. You will be very surprised once you start doing the sums about how much salt you really are consuming a day.

Summary

- By lowering your salt levels and walking 45 minutes briskly per day you could reduce your risk of developing high blood pressure.
- Even if you are currently on blood pressure medications, work with your doctor over a period of time and show that you are committed to coming off these pills for life by making the necessary changes.
- By including wholegrains, fresh fruit and vegetables and lean protein every day in your diet you may find that within a few weeks your blood pressure has reduced.
- Processed foods should only be included once or twice a week as part of a healthy processed and natural diet.

12. Heart Disease

If the pump that is supplying the pressure to send your blood through the miles of blood vessels is not working efficiently then of course it will affect your sex life. Apart from lack of adequate blood flow there are all the other symptoms to cope with which are not necessarily conducive to an unfettered libido.

If you have developed High Blood Pressure and Elevated Cholesterol then you are at risk of developing heart disease. This is a brief overview of some of the heart problems you may be at risk of.

Angina

One of the main causes of angina and heart disease is atherosclerosis.

Atherosclerosis is the hardening of the arteries as a result of plaque that has built up in the arterial walls narrowing the blood vessels and restricting the flow of oxygen rich blood to the heart and other organs such as the brain. Atherosclerosis accounts for almost 75% of deaths from cardiovascular disease.

What Is Angina?

Angina (angina pectoris) is a type of temporary chest pain. There are two types, stable and unstable and both indicate that there is likely to be coronary heart disease.

Stable angina attacks occur after vigorous exercise that requires additional blood to be sent to the heart. An attack might last from one or two minutes to fifteen minutes. Activities that also increase the risk of an attack are cigarette smoking, stress, abrupt changes in temperature or altitude, heavy meals that are not given time to digest and sudden exertion such as running for a bus or up stairs. These types of attack are also described as predictable as they tend to happen between early morning and noon. One reason for this may be the body's inability to go from a state of complete rest to fully active immediately on getting up in the morning. Like an old car it takes time to get all functions working efficiently especially if arteries are blocked and oxygen is in short supply.

Unstable angina is more dangerous as it is also unpredictable and will last longer than fifteen minutes. It can occur at rest and without any previous history of heart disease and should be treated as an emergency as it could indicate that the person is just about to suffer a full heart attack.

What Are the Symptoms of Angina?

People who suffer from angina describe the pain as crushing, burning behind the breastbone and as if there is a weight resting on the chest. The pain can radiate out from the chest and affect the neck, arms, jaw and the abdomen. The person might also feel light headed and experience a faster than normal heartbeat (arrhythmia)

Whether the episode lasts a minute or longer you should seek medical attention. There is a strong possibility that if the attack occurs after eating a very heavy meal that you might be suffering from indigestion. However, if the pain has moved from under your diaphragm and you are experiencing discomfort in any of the other areas that I have mentioned above you should definitely seek medical help.

How Is Angina Diagnosed?

I have already covered high blood pressure and cholesterol as these are the two main indicators that you are at risk of angina. As I already said if you are then put on drugs to lower your blood pressure and cholesterol then these could result in loss of sexual function but should you be suffering from Angina then it is very important that the problem is dealt with as soon as possible and after you have been referred to a specialist and been through a number of tests the extent of the problem will be diagnosed.

This is again why having a regular MOT is so important as both your blood pressure and cholesterol will be measured and if a small increase is identified simple lifestyle changes may be all that is needed.

Should you go to the doctor with symptoms of Angina you may be put through a number of physical tests such as an electrocardiogram (EKG) undergone while you are exercising in a controlled environment, although results can be inconclusive even for patients with extensive heart damage.

Nuclear imaging involves the patient being injected with a radionuclide substance to produce pictures of the heart.

Echocardiogram is a stress test that combined with the EKG can give an image that determines any damage to the heart muscle.

Angiogram is a catheter based test that delivers a special dye that shows up under X-ray and can identify blocked arteries that may be causing the restriction of oxygen to both the heart and other major organs.

What Are the Treatment Options for Angina?

A doctor will ask you for a complete medical history including that of your immediate family and will evaluate the findings of the various tests to determine if you will need a medication or surgery based treatment option.

The medication most commonly prescribed are **Nitrates** such as **nitro-glycerine** that dilate the walls of the blood vessels allowing more blood and therefore oxygen to reach the heart. If there are repeated angina episodes then there could be the addition of **beta-blockers** and **calcium channel blockers**.

- **Beta-blockers** slow the heartbeat and also reduce the strength of the muscle contractions taking some of the load off the organ.
- **Calcium channel blockers** block the entry of calcium into the cells. This dilates the coronary arteries and increases the heart's blood flow.

Antiplatelet and **anticoagulant** drugs inhibit the formation of blood clots by inhibiting the platelets that normal bind together. Aspirin is often prescribed in a relatively low dose, which a patient can take daily. Heparin is one of the more common anticoagulant drugs that is prescribed.

There are a number of surgical options for advanced stages of atherosclerosis and therefore increased angina attacks. These include **angioplasty, stenting and coronary artery bypass grafting.**

- **Angioplasty** is a procedure where a balloon-tipped catheter is inserted in the blocked coronary artery and inflated. The balloon compresses the plaque against the walls of the artery, which increases the blood flow. This is usually combined with the inserting of a stent via the catheter. A stent is a small mesh tube that holds the damaged artery open allowing for increased blood flow.
- A **coronary bypass** is a far more invasive procedure, which involves the grafting of the patient's own veins and arteries from other parts of the body around the damaged blood vessels by passing the blockage.

What Can We Do to Prevent Atherosclerosis and Angina?

One of the most important preventative measures that you can take is to learn about your own body and also the medical history of your immediate family. It is more likely that if your parents, grandparents suffered from heart disease or diabetes then you may also be at a higher risk of the same problems. Diabetes sufferers are more likely to suffer from heart problems and monitoring this through regular blood tests is important if there has been a family history of the disease. Having this knowledge gives you the opportunity to make lifestyle choices that reduce your risk of developing heart disease in your own lifetime.

> *First and foremost,*
> *if you smoke you MUST give up*
> *as this is a major contributor to heart disease.*

Cigarette smoking increases the risk of coronary heart disease by itself. When it acts with other factors, it greatly increases risk. Smoking increases blood pressure, inhibits oxygen uptake during exercise and increases the tendency for blood to clot. Smoking also increases the risk of recurrent coronary heart disease after bypass surgery.

Being overweight puts pressure on your entire body including the heart. When I weighed 330 lbs my resting heart rate was 90 beats a minute instead of the normal 50 to 55. This meant that even at rest my heart was beating 5,400 beats per hour and 129,600 beats per day. My resting heart rate today is 45–50, which is 72,000 beats per day. The result is a 58,000 reduction in the number of times my heart beats in a day or 20,800,000 times a year. The heart is a muscle that suffers wear and tear and by reducing the number of times your heart beats, you are extending the lifetime of this vital organ.

You need to change your diet even if you are on medication for cholesterol and high blood pressure.

Stress is a major contributor to heart disease as the body is producing hormones and other chemicals that put pressure on the heart. Stress also tends to make us reach for what we consider to be de-stresses such as cigarettes, coffee, alcohol and chocolate that either alter our chemical make-up or contribute to arterial damage or weight problems. Certainly the surge of adrenaline caused by severe emotional and physical stress causes the blood to clot more readily, increasing the risk of heart attacks. Adrenaline and its ability to clot blood was only ever meant to be used in a fight or flight reaction to immediate danger and possible harm, not on an everyday basis.

The healthy eating plan for life at the back of the book not only contains the nutrients your body needs to be healthy but also is designed to reduce your risk factors such as High Blood Pressure, Cholesterol and High Blood Sugar.

Arrhythmia

- **Arrhythmia** is an erratic and abnormal heart rate. This is most commonly caused by blocked coronary arteries.
- **Sinus tachycardia** is a regular heartbeat but too fast, usually over 100 beats per minute. It can also be caused by over exertion or stress.
- **Atrial fibrillation** is caused by abnormal electrical activity resulting in heartbeats between 300 to 500 beats per minute.
- **Ventricular tachycardia** is caused by damaged heart muscle resulting in an ineffective heartbeat of between 120–220 beats per minute without the power to push the blood through the system.

Heart Murmurs

We normally cannot hear the blood actually flowing through the heart but sometimes there may be some unusual noises that are called murmurs. These indicate that the smooth flow of blood has become unstable due to structural damage inside the heart. This is quite commonly damage to the valves between the atria and the ventricles either narrowing or leaking.

Heart Valve Disorders

As with any part of the body the heart valves are subject to wear and tear. Our heart function is very dependent on the pumping action and therefore on the health of the valves. There are two types of abnormality, stenosis which is a narrowing of the valve allowing less blood through and an incompetent valve which allows blood to leak back down into the ventricles through an improperly closed valve.

Some valves can be corrected surgically but it is quite common these days to have the valves replaced completely restoring normal heart function. The replacement valves are made from metal and plastic which may require medication to prevent clotting or animal or human tissue which is not as long lasting but does not cause clots.

Heart Attack

A heart attack is probably everyone's worst fear as they get into middle age and it used to be that men over 50 years old were in the highest risk factor. Today men and women alike share that risk and there are an increasing number of younger men and women who are suffering from this potentially fatal heart problem.

A heart attack is also known as a myocardial infarction and involves the death of part of the heart muscle. This is the result of a blockage in the coronary artery, depriving an area of the heart of its oxygen supply.

Usually there will be severe chest pain accompanied by difficulty in breathing, sweating and nausea. If the attack leads to the complete loss of heartbeat then death may occur if prompt treatment is not given.

What Are the Warning Signs of an Impending Heart Attack?
- **Chest discomfort.** Most heart attacks involve discomfort in the centre of the chest that lasts for more than a few minutes, or goes away and comes back. The discomfort can feel like heavy pressure, squeezing of the chest muscles or actual pain.
- **Upper body discomfort.** It is possible for the upper body to be affected with pain or discomfort in one or both arms, the back, neck, jaw and the stomach.

- **Breathing difficulties**. When the chest is tight and painful it is more difficult to take a breath, which is frightening, but you can also experience shortness of breath before any other symptoms occur.
- **Other symptom**s. Cold sweats, nausea and dizziness.

What Do You Do If You Feel That You Are Suffering From a Heart Attack and You Are on Your Own?

One of the first rules if you feel that you are in the beginning phases of a heart attack is not to panic, as this will add to the stress of the situation. I realise that this is easier said than done but there are three things that you can do that will help save your life. You may be experiencing pain and discomfort but you must make every effort to get to a phone.

Contact emergency services tell them you are having a heart attack and give them your address. If at all possible get to the front door and leave it slightly open so that they can gain access.

Take a very deep breath and start to cough as vigorously as possible. Deep breathing gives you oxygen to your lungs and coughing squeezes the heart helping the blood to circulate.

Repeat the deep breath and coughing every two seconds until help arrives or your heart starts to beat normally.

The heart is very difficult to replace and damage to this vital organ is one of the leading causes of death in adults.

It is never too late to change your lifestyle and avoid foods that promote atherosclerosis and eat foods that actively encourage a healthy circulatory system. Making those changes today could possibly save your life.

Summary

- Keeping a regular check on your blood pressure and cholesterol will enable you to reduce your risk of developing heart disease.
- If you exhibit any symptoms of Angina then you need to go to your doctor immediately so that you can undergo tests to eliminate heart disease as the cause. It might be severe indigestion. If however, you don't go and you are worried and stressed about the symptoms this will only add to your risk factors.

13. The Liver

Before I cover cholesterol in the next chapter, it is important that we devote some time to another major organ that is often overlooked as a source of our general health.

The liver is a multi-tasking organ that is capable of around 500 functions. It is also the only organ in the body capable of regenerating itself, provided it has been taken care of and is given the nutrients it needs to be healthy.

However, we live in a modern age with a diet full of preservatives in our processed food, toxins and drugs in the natural food chain, excess sugar, alcohol and lousy fats and keeping our liver functioning well requires attention to both diet and lifestyle.

It would take many books to detail all the workings of the liver so this is merely an overview. We often regard our heart as the most important organ but for me the liver is very high up on the list of reasons to stay healthy.

Where Is the Liver?

The liver sits in the right upper part of the abdomen where it stretches halfway across the left upper abdomen. It is the largest internal organ of the body, weighing between 3 and 4 lbs It is roughly triangular in shape and rests under the right diaphragm and the right lung. Beneath the liver is the gall bladder, attached by the bile duct, and there are blood vessels entering above the liver from the heart called the supra hepatic vena cava carrying

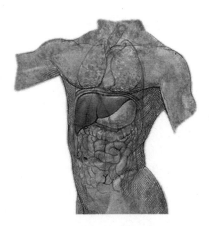

Location of the Liver

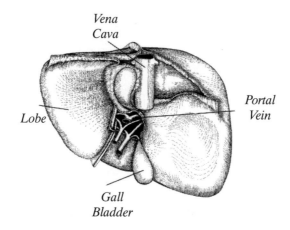

Vena Cava

Portal Vein

Lobe

Gall Bladder

Main parts of the Liver

oxygen rich blood from the heart. It contains veins called the portal system, which take the blood from the intestines to the liver before sending the blood back to the rest of the body.

What Is the Function of the Liver?

The liver has two essential roles, making or processing chemicals and eliminating toxins and waste. Without the portal system none of the nutrients that we have carefully processed and passed into the intestines could be carried in the blood, through the liver, to nourish the body and provide us with energy.

It is not really the liver that does all the work but the millions and millions of cells within the liver that maintain the critical life processes. Specialist cells called hepatocytes deal with the raw materials our body runs on – proteins, carbohydrates and fats.

We are made of protein and we need to consume protein to renew cells and create new ones. It is necessary for the formation of hormones, which are the body's chemical messengers, and also for making enzymes. Unfortunately the body does not necessarily accept all the protein that we consume and it needs to be changed to a format that is usable.

The liver will break down the consumed product and transform it into a protein that the body *does* recognise and can use efficiently. The process involves the raw material being absorbed from the blood in the portal veins into the surrounding hepatocytes where it is synthesised by the enzymes and passed back into the blood.

Any waste however is not re-absorbed into the bloodstream but prepared for elimination.

Carbohydrates are formed from the three essential elements of life, carbon, hydrogen and oxygen. They are most commonly in the form of sugars, which provide us with energy. Our muscles are designed to burn sugar, or sugar like substances, whenever they work. The liver plays a vital role in the process of converting carbohydrates into the appropriate fuels that can be easily accessed by the muscles.

It does this by converting carbohydrates into two forms very similar to pure sugar. One is used for a quick fix and the other is put into storage for later use. The instant energy comes from *glucose* and the stored *glycogen*. A lack of sugar as fuel can lead to brain damage. The body being the survivor it is, makes sure that there is sufficient stored to provide us with energy when we need it, such as in the case of running from a rampaging bull or if we are faced with starvation.

The balance is critical, and a healthy liver will ensure that there is just enough sugar in the blood at all times.

Fats are not always the bad guys. We know that there are good fats and bad fats but the body does need fat for insulation and as a shock absorber to surround major organs. The liver turns the fat we eat into forms that can be built into or renew existing fatty tissue. Some of us have a little more of that than we might wish but it is our storehouse and vital to our wellbeing.

Finally, the liver ensures that waste products, both in the form of toxins that have found their way into the body and from by-products resulting from the thousands of chemical processes that are taking place throughout the body every minute of the day, are disposed of correctly

The waste disposal cells are called Kuppfer cells, after the man who discovered them. They are the Dyson's of the cell fraternity, sucking up bacteria and toxins before handing them over to the hepatocytes for processing.

When you suffer from either the common cold or influenza, the liver works as part of the immune system to weaken or destroy these harmful germs. This is why following the healthy eating plan which is nutrient packed can have such a tremendous effect on your general health, particularly in the winter months when there are so many more infections around.

An example of a toxic by-product is the ammonia produced during the breakdown of protein. It is poisonous, and the liver cells neutralise it sending the harmless waste, in the form of urea, back into the bloodstream. This applies to alcohol, medication or drugs so it is vitally important that your liver is functioning at an optimum level for your health and survival.

What Other Roles Does the Liver Carry Out?

The liver stores iron as well as other vitamins and minerals that you need, such as Vitamin B12.

Bilirubin is an orange-yellow waste product of red blood cells that can be toxic in large amounts in your body and can cause conditions like yellow jaundice. The liver excretes this bilirubin into the small bowel where bacteria can change it into the safer green coloured biliverdin.

The liver also makes clotting factors that stop bleeding after injury, and without which you could bleed to death.

The liver helps manage the cholesterol in our body – and the body *needs* cholesterol – but like anything in excess it can do more harm than good. It forms the base molecule for hormones like oestrogen and testosterone, and it is also the base for bile acids that are used to emulsify fat in the small bowel so that fat and fat soluble vitamins like E and K can be absorbed. Because Cholesterol is so vital to our hormonal functions you will find more information in the next chapter.

Do Diet and Lifestyle Play That Much of a Role In Liver Health?

Well, think about everything that you put into your mouth and the changes it will go through before eventually leaving your body. I think of the liver as the guardian of my health because of all the complex processes it is in charge of, that ensure that I am not only nourished but am also protected from germs and toxins.

The saying "We are what we eat" is never more true as is "You are only as good as what you eat". If you have adopted a diet strategy which involves eating high fat, processed, sugar laden and nutritionally sterile foods, you cannot expect your liver to transform it into the ultimate wonder diet. It can only work with what you give it and if you add excessive alcohol consumption into the equation, you will find that the liver can become overwhelmed, and will suffer damage.

The good news is that the liver regenerates extremely quickly provided it does not have scarred tissue. Within a matter of 6 weeks you can improve your liver health and therefore you general health quite dramatically.

Cirrhosis of the Liver

Because the liver is such a complex organ there are over 100 diseases that can affect its health.

However, around 90% of liver damage is caused by alcoholic hepatitis or viral infections such as *Hepatitis A* and *Hepatitis B*. *Hepatitis A* is transmitted from contaminated food and water. It results in fever and sickness and a yellowing of the skin and whites of the eye called jaundice, a condition that lasts approximately three weeks.

There is a much more dangerous 'serum hepatitis' called *Hepatitis B*, which is also a viral infection – but this is spread by sexual intercourse and the use of infected needles or contaminated blood products. It results in headaches, intermittent fevers and chills, extreme fatigue and jaundice. It can take up to six months for the symptoms to appear and recovery can be very slow and is often unsuccessful.

Some diseases of the liver are hereditary and are usually diagnosed in a baby or young toddler. These include Alagille syndrome, Alpha 1-Antitrypsin deficiency, Autoimmune hepatitis, the result of an abnormal immune system at birth, Galactosemia, Wilson's disease – the abnormal storage of copper – and Haemochromatosis – the abnormal storage of iron.

One of the dangers of long term medication is that, like everything else we ingest, the medication also needs to go through the liver to be processed. This also applies to extensive exposure to chemicals in a home or work environment. Both are likely to overwork the liver and cause damage.

It is obvious that hereditary conditions and viral infections require treatment by medical experts. What we are concerned with is the general health of the liver to prevent damage and to improve function by making some adjustments to our lifestyles.

What Is Cirrhosis of the Liver?

Cirrhosis occurs when scar tissue replaces dead or injured liver cells. It is caused by disease, or more commonly alcoholism. The scarring distorts the normal structure and re-growth of liver cells and the flow of blood through the liver, from the intestines, is blocked. This restricts the functions carried out by the liver, such as processing proteins or toxins. This in turn can lead to other medical problems such as gallstones, toxicity and fluid retention in the legs and abdomen. Because the liver produces proteins that help clot the blood, damage can lead to excessive or prolonged bleeding – both internally and from cuts and injuries.

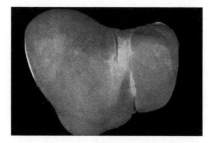

Normal Liver

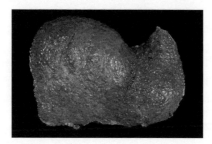

Liver with Cirrhosis

There is no cure for cirrhosis but the spread of the scarring can be stopped, and improvement in the health of the liver achieved in most cases, if the original cause of the damage is removed: For example, by stopping drinking alcohol.

An even more frightening finding is that more and more teenagers and young adults are presenting with cirrhosis of the liver. *The cause is not excessive alcohol but excessive consumption of soft drinks containing sugars, acid and artificial sweeteners.*

How Do We Help the Liver Cope With Everyday Pressures?

The most obvious place to start is with the amount of alcohol that we drink. One of the myths surrounding cirrhosis is that you have to be a chronic alcoholic to get the disease but you do not have to go to this extreme to damage your liver. The good news is that alcoholic hepatitis does not necessarily lead to cirrhosis of the liver, and certainly not to the extent where a transplant is required. It can take many years of dedicated drinking to reach that stage, but that will depend on the person.

No one person is the same and I often quote the saying "one man's meat is another man's poison". We are all unique and this applies to our internal operating systems as well. I am sure that we have been to parties and watched one person have two glasses of wine and be as drunk as a lord and someone else down drink after drink without any apparent affect. That is to say that from the outside they look okay but of course their liver may be telling a different story.

Like many internal organs, the liver has a primary purpose in life and that is for the host body to survive. It will struggle daily to cope with excessive stress and harmful contaminants and it is often only when it is in the final stages of disease that we see the external evidence for ourselves.

Generally speaking, drinking more than two or three drinks per day is going to affect your liver to some degree. Binge drinking at the weekend is something we are all guilty of from time to time. We do not have a drink all week and then on the weekend we go out for a meal or have friends around enjoying pre-dinner drinks and a few glasses of wine followed by a couple or more liqueurs. This is bingeing as far as your liver is concerned, particularly if it is accompanied by a rich meal full of fats and proteins that require processing.

The liver, like the rest of the body, needs antioxidants to prevent oxidative damage. A diet high in processed foods is not only going to give the liver even more work to do, processing additives and excess chemicals such as phosphorus, but is also *not* going to give it the raw materials it requires for its own health.

Even if we do *not* drink we can still cause damage to our liver by having a very high-fat diet. The liver again is overworked and often underpaid. Healthy fats play a very important role in our diet but they still need to be consumed in moderation. Remember that everything you eat has to be processed and if you overwhelm the digestive system and the liver with high quantities of food that it considers to be a toxin it will be overwhelmed and the system and process will break down.

The current trend of excluding all carbohydrates in favour of high-fat diets is not healthy for the liver, or the kidneys. The biggest problem is that people succeed for the first couple of weeks in losing weight and then stay on the regime for far too long, leading to liver function problems.

What Are Some of the Simple Ways We Can Modify Our Diet and Lifestyle to Help Our Liver?

First, keep an alcohol diary for a few weeks. Look at your drinking patterns and be realistic about exactly how much you are consuming. If you are drinking two bottles of wine per week make sure that it is spread out through the seven days rather than all on one night.

If you drink spirits such as whisky, how many bottles are you getting through a week and would you drink less if you changed some environmental factors?

Drinking is a habit. The sun is over the yardarm and we reach for that first glass of wine of the evening. We sit in front of the television and have a whisky and water or two before or after dinner. We go out for lunch or dinner and automatically ask for the wine list.

Just to give you a little incentive to modify the amount you drink you can refer to the "Fat Accumulation Table". A bottle of wine per night equates to over *60 lbs* in body fat a year.

So, if you are in the habit of sharing a bottle every night you may have an explanation for the extra *30 lbs* you are carrying around.

Drinking, as part of a healthy eating plan, is fine as long as you don't eat less so that you can still enjoy your two glasses of wine per night. Also on that point, there are many differences in the sizes of glasses we are talking about. *Goblets that hold half a bottle of wine do **not** count for one glass!*

Reducing your alcohol intake will benefit you in other ways too. You will have more energy and skin, hair and eyes will look great.

The other area to look at is your fat intake. Keep a food diary along with your alcohol diary for a week and some simple adjustments will make considerable changes to your fat intake.

- Do avoid using low fat alternatives as the additives and hydrogenated fat are more than harmful enough in their own right. Have red meat by all means once or twice a week but the rest of the time use chicken, turkey, salmon, white fish and even vegetarian options.
- Skimmed milk and buttermilk have less fat but still contain nutrients and there are plenty of options for healthy yoghurts.
- Use cheese like Edam instead of full fat cheddar but use moderately.
- Make your own salad dressings and mayonnaise using olive oil and low fat yoghurts.
- Grill, bake, poach and steam chicken, meat and fish whenever possible.
- One area that is full of fat and additives is salted snacks. So with your one or two glasses of wine per night, enjoy vegetable strips with home-made dip and dried fruit and nuts.

The Cholesterol Link to Our Overall Health

A vital factor involved in the health of most of our major organs is a substance in our bodies called cholesterol. For example the extremely common lifestyle and age related medical condition high blood pressure that I covered in the health of our circulatory system, is the result of an imbalance in the Cholesterol circulating in your bloodstream. As you will have read in the chapter on brain health and in following chapters on the heart and circulatory system it can directly affect the function of major organs and systems. However, the current trend of prescribing Statins to lower cholesterol can also have an adverse effect. On you sex life. As you will read in the next chapter – Cholesterol is essential in the production of hormones, including those that maintain a healthy sex life.

14. The Cholesterol Link to High Blood Pressure and the Effect of Statins on Your Sex Life

What Is Cholesterol?

Good question! Doctors and therapists bandy about terms that have little or no meaning for many of us. They use terms like LDL and HDL and the ratio to each other and how this affects our blood and that we may therefore at risk of having a stroke or a heart attack.

Cholesterol is waxy fat that is present in all of us. The liver manufactures around 80% of the Cholesterol in our body and the other 20% is ingested in the food that we eat. Most Cholesterol that we eat is from animal products such as meat, eggs and dairy products.

Cholesterol on its own has no way of moving through the bloodstream so is carried along by proteins called apoliproteins. These proteins wrap around Cholesterol and other fats in the form of packages that are called lipoproteins.

There are four different lipoproteins:
- **HDL** (High-density lipoproteins or Healthy Cholesterol)
- **LDL** (Low-Density lipoproteins or Lousy Cholesterol)
- **VLDL** (Very low density lipoproteins or Very Lousy Cholesterol) and finally
- **Chylomicrons**, which carry a very small percentage of Cholesterol but which, are very rich in a type of fat called triglycerides.

Why Do We Have Cholesterol?

Cholesterol and triglycerides are important as building blocks in the structure of cells and also in the production of hormones and energy. As I have mentioned the amount in our bodies is largely dependent on the liver and to a lesser degree the cholesterol we ingest in our food. Without cholesterol in our system we would not have any sex hormones, which is why we are going to be spending some time with the latest 'miracle' drug called statins.

Food, like our own bodies, has LDL and HDL and that is where changes in our diet and eating the right kind of fats can promote HDL in our own systems. HDL works by reducing the cholesterol in our tissues and taking it back to the liver for reprocessing. This protects the tissues in the lining of the arteries from hardening. So the higher the HDL the lower the artery disease

I have already covered atherosclerosis, which is hardening of the arteries, which in turn leads to High Blood pressure and coronary disease. When this happens, a person generally has very high levels of LDL or VLDL. Conversely people whose blood measures high levels of HDL or the High-Density lipoproteins have little or no hardening of the arteries or evidence of heart disease. HDL has been proven to reduce the levels of LDL in the blood so it should be a significant part of our Healthy Eating programme.

The lifestyle challenge is to ensure that the balance of LDL and HDL is correct so that excessive LDL does not lead to damage and clogging of our arteries.

How Can You Tell If You Have High Cholestorol?

I think that like many internal problems that we accumulate as we get older, cholesterol is another silent killer. It is not visible on the outside and you may only know you have a problem when you develop arterial or heart problems.

It is a very simple test that can take five minutes in your local pharmacy. A blood sample is taken after the person being tested has fasted for several hours. For example the easiest thing to do is not to have anything to eat after 6.00 pm and have your test early the next morning before you eat breakfast.

A mole is a measurement of molecules. The unit is modified by either a milli or a micro or some other prefix and the measurement for Cholesterol is mmol/l (millimoles/litre). Alternatively, if you were having a test for blood glucose it would be measured in mg/dl which is milligrams per decilitre.

For our purposes:
- Average Cholesterol is 5.7 mmol/l
- Ideal Cholesterol is 5 mmol/l
- Mildly Elevated Cholesterol is between 5 and 6.4 mmol/l
- Moderately Elevated Cholesterol is between 6.5 and 7.8 mmol/l
- Very High Cholesterol levels would be above 7.8 mmol/l

These measurements are however affected by the different levels of LDL and HDL within the blood sample and taking into account some other arterial and heart disease risks such as smoking, high blood pressure or diabetes. It is therefore possible that someone has a high total level of Cholesterol but because there are very few risk factors or a high level of HDL, they are less likely to develop future health problems.

If you already have problems and particularly if high Cholesterol runs in your family, then you should ideally keep your Cholesterol below the 5 mmol/l mark – this means keeping the LDL measurement at a lower level too. Certainly below 3 mmol/l.

What Do You Do If You Have a Test Result That Indicates That not Only Do You Have Elevated Cholesterol but Your LDL Is Also High?

Well it is important not to panic. If you have done a test at a pharmacy then go to your doctor with the result and talk to him about your current lifestyle. Depending on the level of the test result, he may be happy for you to make changes to your lifestyle and diet in the first instance before prescribing cholesterol reducing drugs.

If your test is borderline, then you need to sit down and work out how you are going to make changes that will affect your next test, which I suggest you carry out in 6 weeks time.

The first step is to take a good, hard look at your current lifestyle and diet. For two or three days write down *everything* that you eat, drink and any exercise that you do. Pay particular attention to the fats in your diet. Although 80% of our Cholesterol is manufactured in our liver, a diet very high in the wrong sorts of fat can increase our Cholesterol levels significantly and one of the things we need to do now is identify which are unhealthy fats and which are those that will benefit you.

Are There Any Other Factor That May Affect Your Cholesterol Levels?

Cholesterol problems can run in families. If it is inherited it is called Familial Hypercholesterolaemia or Familial Hyperlipidaemia, which is where the triglyceride level is very high too. Other diseases may also affect your Cholesterol levels such as diabetes or kidney disease. Your alcohol intake can also have a bearing on your levels.

What Is the Difference Between Good and Bad Fats?

There can be some confusion about fats and if they are good or bad. Should you eat butter or low fat spread? Do Avocados cause high Cholesterol?

First off, let's take a look at the fats you are likely to encounter in your everyday diet.

There are two BAD Fats

- **Saturated Fats**, which raise your total, blood Cholesterol as well as the LDL, which is the lousy Cholesterol. These are mainly found in animal products, some seafood and some plants.
- **Tran's fats** are manufactured fats by scientists to put into our processed food products. Liquid oil is hydrogenated to extend its shelf life but in the process Trans fatty acids are formed. These are found in most processed foods including margarine. Most fast food is full of Tran's fats, as are snacks such as microwave popcorn.

The GOOD Fats are

- **Monounsaturated fats**, which lower total Cholesterol and LDL and increase the HDL. Contained in nuts, like the walnuts on our Superfood list, and olive oil.
- **Polyunsaturated fats** also lower total Cholesterol and LDL Cholesterol and these would come from Salmon, Soya, and sunflower oils – Omega-3 fatty acids that I covered in a previous chapter.

If you look at my list of 'superfoods' you will find that many of the foods on the list either contain monounsaturated or polyunsaturated fats and will help reduce your total Cholesterol level and also improve the ratio between the LDL and the HDL.

Should We Cut Out Fats Altogether From Our Diets?

Absolutely not. Our bodies are designed to use fats for a number of processes that are essential to our health and well being. Fats assist in the absorption of nutrients. They keep our nervous system healthy and maintain our cell membranes. It is, as I have always said, when you have too much of a good thing that the processes break down and the body suffers damage. It is about knowing what is good for us and what is bad for us.

Taking in too much fat causes obesity, heart disease and some types of cancers. It is about understanding the role of fats in our health and making informed decisions about what you will and will not eat that is crucial to your general health and specific problems such as sexual dysfunction.

You control how much processed food you put in your mouth. No one is actually force feeding you nor are they making you eat margarine instead of butter or using hydrogenated fats for cooking instead of butter. Take a good look again at what you are eating and tick anything that has hydrogenated fats in them. If any doubt check with the section at the back of the book on dangerous additives in our foods.

How Do We Live Life To the Full When We Restrict Ourselves From Eating Any Foods That Have Bad Fats in Them?

The answer is that you don't restrict these foods completely. What would be the point? You would not last a week.

I have said before that I believe in the 80/20 rule. If 80% of the time you are following the healthy eating plan – then it will not do you a great deal of harm to have the occasional bad fat.

The really good thing is that your Cholesterol level is not like a rollercoaster, affected by every single meal of item of food. It is your overall diet that you are living with those effects your levels. That means that you can still go out from time to time and have a large steak and chips. Particularly if you are already following the activity plan we talked about too.

Exercise plays a large part in controlling your Cholesterol levels. Don't forget that your body, if it is processing and metabolising food correctly, as it should, will be using all foods to provide energy. And if you are taking a brisk 45-minute walk each day, you will be using some of the higher-fat foods to provide you with fuel.

What Projects Should We Be Putting in Place to Ensure That Our Cholesterol Levels Are Where They Should Be?

Project One

It would be better, in my opinion, to have a scrape of pure butter than a larger portion of Tran's fatty acids. There are some spreads that claim to reduce Cholesterol. I personally don't use them but some people swear by them. That is your decision. If you are having more butter or spread than bread or toast then halve it.

Project Two

Change your cooking oil to either Olive Oil or Sunflower Oil. Do not deep-fry but use the smallest amount possible to grease the pan.

Project Three

Instead of putting butter on your vegetables use a dribble of seasoned olive oil. The same for eating your bread in restaurants. In Mediterranean countries olive oil is put on the table to have with your bread for a very good reason. It is healthier for you.

Project Four

Whatever recipes you use – look for creative ways to reduce the fat in them. Make sure that if you use mince, for example, that you buy the top quality, which is usually 100% pure beef without fillers. If you like steak then buy lean cuts rather than fatty ones. When cooking, instead of extra fat, use broths to prevent the meat from sticking.

Project Five

Find alternatives for your salty and high fat snacks. If you really cannot do without nuts with your evening drink then start eating walnuts, or other unsalted nuts like brazils, that contain healthy fat. You still need to watch how many you are eating, as they will add to your total fat content. Avoid crisps and other prepared snacks, as they are full of Trans fatty acids.

Project Six

Think about balance. You can have high Cholesterol but if the ratio of HDL to LDL is good then you are at less risk of causing artery problems. So make sure that if you are having an occasional piece of cheese in your diet that it is counteracted with some of the good fat items such as Avocados, walnuts, salmon, green tea, brown rice, oats, oranges, onions, garlic, turkey. The same applies to eggs. Having an egg for breakfast each morning is not a problem if the rest of your diet contains foods that help balance the Cholesterol.

Project seven

Check your labels. Look at the fat content of some of the foods that you are eating on a regular basis and you may be horrified by the total amount of fat that you are ingesting without even knowing it. You may have assumed that you had a healthy diet. In some cases you may be vegetarian and have bought processed foods thinking they were healthy. Unfortunately not all are.

Statins and the Link To Sexual Performance

There are times when medication is essential and it is accepted that there are men who require drugs such as Viagra to enjoy a normal sex life following illness or surgery. There are also people who suffer from the hereditary form of cholesterol that rarely responds to lifestyle changes and taking medication is necessary.

In recent months it has been advocated that every man over the age of 50 should automatically be put on statins to prevent heart disease in later life.

I have never heard anything so criminally absurd in my life. My frustration with the blanket prescription of medication rather than establishing the causes of conditions such as blood pressure and cholesterol levels is limitless.

These conditions are lifestyle related in the majority of cases and are the result of poor diet, smoking and alcohol. But, do we hand out a diet sheet and instructions to come back in six months? Of course not because we do not have the time to educate patients about their bodies and how they work, we do not have the time to explain that they need to eat a better diet including how all the nutrients work and so we find it easier to write a prescription for a drug that might do the job.

However, that drug will have side effects and in the long term we do not know the effects on our general health by taking something that has to pass through our body affecting every process on the way.

One of the most important side effects of taking a cholesterol lowering drug is that your sex hormones will be affected.

Cholesterol is the precursor for the steroid hormones which determine our sexuality, control the reproductive process and is the sole source for our sex hormones androgen, oestrogen and progesterone.

*There have been many reports from patients on statins over the years of **loss of sex drive and erectile dysfunction** but it is only recently that research has confirmed that the reduction of cholesterol in your system is directly related to the medication.*

So, what happens when a high percentage of men over 50 are given statins automatically?

Well one thing is for sure and that is a high percentage may not have elevated cholesterol and therefore the statins will reduce normal levels to below safe levels.

This will result in a great many more men experiencing sexual dysfunction.

This brings me to the women who are already feeling below par because of hormonal changes in their 40's and 50's. Chances are that those with elevated cholesterol will have been put on statins and may be wondering where their already depleted sex drive has gone.

This is just one of the side effects of taking this drug. If you are currently taking statins and have been suffering from unexplained muscle pains, depression or nerve damage then you need to talk to your doctor about your prescription. Again I stress that I do not advocate taking yourself off medication without consulting your doctor but there is a better way to lower dietary related elevated cholesterol and it does not involve taking a pill.

Summary

- Most people who suffer from elevated cholesterol could lower it by making dietary changes and taking moderate exercise.
- Taking pills for the rest of your life rather than making those changes is not just lazy it could ultimately be harmful for you and may well affect your sex life.
- Food does not have to taste bland and you certainly should not stop eating all fats as they are an important addition to our daily diet. Just identify the good fats to eat.

- Without a normal level of cholesterol in the body the sex hormones will not be produced efficiently leading to some level of sexual dysfunction.
- You can reduce your cholesterol in six weeks by making some basic and simple changes to your lifestyle.

15. The Diabetes Link to Poor Sexual Performance

What Exactly Is Diabetes?

Diabetes is a set of related diseases in which the body cannot regulate the amount of sugar (glucose) in the blood.

Glucose is what gives you energy. Without it you would be unable to complete many every day to day tasks let alone exercise or lead any kind of active lifestyle.

The liver produces glucose from our diet. We have a number of hormones which normally regulate the level of glucose in our blood, one of which is insulin. We have a small organ that produces insulin and other enzymes that help us digest our foods and extract the nutrients.

This organ is the pancreas and whilst people are more familiar with the major organs such as the heart, liver and kidneys they tend to know less about these little organs that actually have a vital role in keeping us fit and healthy.

The Pancreas is an elongated, tapered organ across the abdomen and the stomach. The widest part rests in the curve of the duodenum which is the first part of the small intestine – the tapered part ends near the spleen.

The organ is made up of two types of tissue – Exocrine and Endocrine. The exocrine tissue secretes the digestive enzymes that help break down the carbohydrates, proteins and fats in the duodenum. The enzymes travel down the pancreatic duct into the bile duct inactive – they then pass into the duodenum where they are activated and start working on the food that has arrived there.

Another important function of the exocrine tissue is the secretion of bicarbonate, which neutralises the stomach acid, which is very important, as it is so strong.

The endocrine tissues secrete the hormones including insulin as well as glucagon, which regulate the level of glucose in the blood. It is the malfunction of this secretion, which causes diabetes.

Without insulin the glucose has no access to the parts of our body that utilise fuel such as the liver, muscles and fat cells.

What Are the Different Types of Diabetes?

There are two common types of diabetes.

- **Type 1** Diabetes means that a person cannot manufacture sufficient insulin from the pancreas for glucose management.
- **Type 2** Diabetes is where, although there is insulin, the body is unable to use it properly, which means that the glucose again is not used efficiently.

  Sometimes people can be suffering from both a lack of insulin and then the inability to use what they do produce.

- **Type 1** Diabetes is the rarer of the two. It is often diagnosed in childhood or teens. It is commonly called insulin dependent diabetes. Usually it is because the body has either never produced sufficient insulin or has stopped producing it altogether for some reason.
- **Type 1** can also be found in older patients due to factors such as too much alcohol, disease or the removal of the pancreas.
- Type 1 patients usually have to be treated daily with insulin to maintain sufficient levels to manage the glucose and therefore their energy levels.
- **Type 2** diabetes has a much stronger genetic link and a great deal of research is currently going on to identify the exact gene. There are a number of lifestyle factors, which also increase the risk of getting Type 2 as we get older. Being overweight, not getting any exercise, taking in too much sugar in the diet, drinking too much and also ageing – the risk increases significantly over the age of 65. This is why this is more commonly called late onset diabetes. Type 2 diabetes is by far the most common and accounts for over 90% of diabetics. The good news is that **Type 2** responds very positively to diet and lifestyle changes and following a balanced diet with regular exercise can significantly reduce the need for medication.

There is also a third type of diabetes which is temporary and that occurs during pregnancy.

Who Is Most at Risk of Developing Type 2 Diabetes?

Some of the risk factors for developing Type 2 diabetes are also common to many of the age-related problems we have already looked at. High blood pressure, high cholesterol, high fat diet, being overweight and not doing any exercise. These all put enormous pressure on the body systems -the pancreas being part of that system.

It is estimated that millions of men and women have a condition called pre-diabetes where they have all the markers including high blood sugar but it has not become full-blown diabetes. Combine this pre-disposition with elevated blood pressure and unhealthy cholesterol and you have a recipe for not only potentially life threatening conditions but also a decrease in sexual performance.

The good news is that like high blood pressure and elevated cholesterol levels, blood sugar can be stabilised by following a balanced diet and exercise programme.

As I have mentioned before, if your doctor confirms that you have high blood sugar and suggests taking medication, work with him or her to change your lifestyle first if possible and then retest in a few weeks to determine if the risk has been reduced.

At the back of the book is the healthy eating plan for life which will reduce the amount of sugar you are taking in and reduce your risk of developing diabetes as you get older.

I would suggest that you get tested before you begin the programme and then six weeks later. If you are concerned by the first reading then please do consult a doctor.

What Sort of Symptoms Might Indicate a Pre-Diabetic or Diabetic Condition?

Type 1 diabetes as we have already said usually is detected in childhood or adolescence often when the child has suffered a viral attack or an injury.

Some of the symptoms they might experience are:
• nausea, vomiting, chronic fatigue and dehydration

Type 2, which is the most common, can have subtle symptoms that we can miss for years. It may not be detected until a check up for blood pressure when e.g eye problems may be noticed.

The most common symptoms for anyone to look out for are the following:

Extreme Fatigue. Remember that we said that the energy from glucose is ineffective. It is not being distributed to the necessary systems and so the body switches over to using fat partially or completely. Burning fat at that rate takes up a great deal of energy itself causing the person to feel very tired all the time.

Weight Loss. Because of the problems with the pancreas food is not processed efficiently leading to lack of nutrients. Calories are also not processed efficiently along with the nutrients so although someone may appear to eat a great deal and have a very healthy diet, they don't get the calories or nutrients and lose weight.

Combine this with the thermogenic effect of the body burning fat instead of glucose and you have extreme weight loss.

Excessive Thirst. High blood sugar levels cause the body to send a signal to the brain to dilute the blood, which translates into thirst. The body encourages more water consumption to dilute the high blood sugar level back to normal. You might experience this in a temporary way if you have had too much wine to drink and then find yourself drinking glasses of water through the night and the next morning. Alcohol is sugar and too much in the bloodstream causes that same message to be sent to the brain.

Excessive urination. Another way that the body tries to get rid of the excess sugar is through the urine. So going to the loo a lot is an indication that there might be something wrong. This leads to more dehydration as of course water leaves the body as well as sugar, this sends more signals to the brain to drink more and it becomes a vicious circle.

Increased Hunger. Although a person suffering from diabetes will usually lose weight, they will find that their hunger increases and making them eat far more than they would normally.

To try and deal with the excess sugar in the blood the pancreas will secrete more insulin – excess insulin stimulates hunger.

Slow-to-heal Wounds. High sugar levels prevent the white blood cells, which are a vital part of the immune system from doing their job. They are weakened and unable to deal with the bacteria that damages tissues and cells so wounds are very slow to heal causing open sores which appear particularly on the legs and heels of the feet.

Yeast Infections is the other problem. This links a yeast and fungal condition called Candida Albicans, the subject of the next chapter. The yeast gets a hold because the immune system is repressed and its main food source is of course yeast and sugar so it thrives and causes skin infections, thrush and cystitis. Candida is also a common cause of reproductive and sexual dysfunction and because it is rarely diagnosed correctly, remains untreated. It is estimated that over 65% of the population of the western world suffers from an overgrowth of Candida.

Elevated blood sugar levels can cause the retina to be damaged so one of the symptoms of a diabetic condition is *Blurry Vision*. As this can be an early symptom it is always a good idea to have your blood sugar levels tested and to talk to the doctor about the results.

Fluctuating blood sugar levels cause a number of **depressive states**:

- Irritability
- loss of memory
- confusion and
- extreme lethargy

can occur in varying degrees. It is very important that if you are talking to someone and they seem to have all these symptoms and be disorientated and dazed that you get them medical help as quickly as possible as they could lapse into a diabetic coma.

What Happens if Diabetes Is not Treated?

If the problem is not treated, over time there can be some complications that affect the rest of your body.

Long term elevated blood sugar levels – called Hyperglycaemia – can lead to damage to the eyes, kidneys, nerves and blood vessels.

One of the leading causes of blindness in the elderly is diabetic retinopathy. This is where the retina is damaged completely.

It can cause kidney failure, damage to the nerves which can result in leg ulcers. Also nerves in the stomach which can lead to stomach and intestinal problems. The body suddenly seems unable to control heart rate and blood pressure as the system comes under increased pressure.

Diabetes is also connected to heart problems. Diabetes causes fatty plaques inside arteries, which leads to clots that can lead to strokes. High blood pressure and cholesterol levels increase causing more damage to blood vessels. This in turn of course leads to damaged blood vessels in the penis and will affect its ability to achieve and maintain an erection.

The last thing that you should do if you are suffering from blood vessel damage is take a stimulant such as Viagra to obtain an erection as you could cause further damage and possibly blood loss.

Does Changing Your Lifestyle Make a Difference?

The great thing is that it is never too late. Particularly with Type 2 diabetes.

Even with Type 1, following a sensible diet can make a difference to your overall health.

Firstly it is a very simple thing to **go and get your blood sugar levels tested**. My own local pharmacy does a test in five minutes that tells you not only your blood sugar levels but also blood pressure and cholesterol. You can expand that test according to your requirements.

If you have any worries that you might be at risk, then take a test and then at least you know where you stand. Many of us have elevated sugar levels that are not causing diabetes but are a nudge for us to take a look at our lifestyle and moderate it so that the risk factors are reduced.

A healthy diet and lifestyle can help prevent the onset of diabetes. Even if you do have diabetes, once under the care of a doctor and monitored medication, then a change in lifestyle can over a period of months result in a reduction of the medication and in some cases patients have been able to stop it altogether.

Having said that, of course, as always, you must never change any medication that you have been prescribed if you have not first consulted your doctor.

Because of the risk factors involved in having a diet very high in refined sugars I am devoting a complete chapter (Ch. 18) to the substance itself.

Summary

- Sugar, white flour products and lots of white animal fats are called the "white death" and there is a reason for that – they clog your arteries and cause blood sugar problems. You do not need to remove sugar entirely but you well be obtaining natural sugars from any fruits and some vegetables that you eat. Manuka Honey which is anti-bacterial and anti-viral can be included in small amounts because it is strong and it is healthy. Our bodies have been processing honey for almost as long as we have been around.
- Check your labels – the maximum sugar you should be consuming per day in total is 10 level teaspoons. You will be surprised how much sugar there is in a bowl of cereal – pasta sauce – chocolate bar even before you put spoons of sugar in your tea. Get in the habit of looking at your labels – it could save reduce not just your risk of developing diabetes but also sexual dysfunction.

16. Do You Have Candida Albicans?

It is estimated that Candida Albicans affects an estimated 65% of the population of the western world. It certainly was one of the root causes behind my own obesity problem and was clearly a factor in the health of the majority of clients that I have worked with.

The reason for including it in this book on sexual dysfunction is fundamental. There are over 120 symptoms connected to Candida which cause many conditions including reproductive, hormonal problems and obesity. I suggest that you complete the questionnaire on the following pages and if your score is in the highest bracket you may have found a contributory factor to your sexual problems.

What Is Candida Albicans?

Candida Albicans is a yeast, which inhabits all humans, usually only in small amounts. It is also known as Monilia, Thrush, Candidiasis and Yeast Infection. In its natural, mild form it is harmless and is simply part of the soup of bacteria that inhabits our intestines.

The basic precondition for a fungal disease is an impaired immune system. This can be the result of an illness, over-use of antibiotics, intensive dieting over a long period of time and recurring infections. Latterly there has been considerable research into why women who have never had anti-biotics are developing Candida Albicans in their late 20's and 30's and again in their 50's. The answer seems to be that the birth control pill and HRT both hormone altering drugs are having a similar effect as anti-biotics.

Look at antibiotics for instance. In most cases antibiotics are broad spectrum not specific. Because, without a lab test it is difficult to tell the specific strain of bacteria responsible for an infection, the use of broad spectrum drugs usually guarantees that the bacteria in question will be killed off. Unfortunately, like chemotherapy not only the bad bacteria are killed off but also the good bacteria in your body. Your intestine, which has a very fragile balance of good and bad bacteria, is vulnerable and this is where Candida Albicans can start to take over your intestinal tract.

What Happens To the Candida Bacteria That Make It Harmful?

If Candida yeast is allowed to grow unchecked, it changes from its normal yeast fungal form to a mycelial-fungal form that produces rhizoids. These long root-like components are capable of piercing the walls of the digestive tract and breaking down the protective barriers between the intestines and the blood. This breakthrough allows many allergens to enter the bloodstream causing allergic reactions. Mucus is also formed around major organs and in the lining of the stomach. This prevents your digestive system from functioning efficiently. The result is poorly digested foods and wasted nutrients. Your body begins to suffer a deficiency of these nutrients and it leads to chronic fatigue.

What Are The Symptoms of a Candida Overgrowth?

The most common of the allergic reactions are:
- Watering, tearing or dry eyes.
- Itchy inner ears and dry throats that come and go.
- A dripping and itchy nose.
- Unexplained rashes.

These symptoms are almost always accompanied by a craving for either bread or savoury snacks such as crisps or for sweets in the form of chocolate particularly. Sometimes clients tell me that they have not got a sweet tooth and don't eat chocolate, but when I read their food diary, I soon spot the biscuits, cakes and alcohol that are eaten or drunk every day.

Let me give you an idea of some of the complaints you could be suffering from that are directly related to Candida Albicans.

- Fatigue – people who are suffering from Chronic Fatigue Syndrome or ME test positive for Candida.
- Numbness, burning or tingling in your fingers or hands.
- Insomnia.
- Abdominal pain.
- Constipation or diarrhoea.

- Bloating and especially Irritable Bowel Syndrome.
- Thrush and urinary tract infections
- Sexual dysfunction and loss of sexual drive.
- Depression and panic attacks are common symptoms as is shaking or getting very irritable when hungry.
- Some people suffer from unexplained muscle or joint pains and are often diagnosed with arthritis.
- Candida bacteria are a parasite and like all parasites it will take the nourishment meant for you and you will then suffer from a depressed immune system.
- Headaches and mood swings.
- Chronic rashes or hives and you will be more prone to food intolerances that cause discomfort or some form of physical symptom.
- The most significant problem is the strain which all of the toxins place on the liver. This can result in chronic fatigue, discomfort and depression.
- The list is virtually endless – which just adds to the confusion at the time of diagnosis
- To kill off the overgrowth you will need to eat a fresh and unprocessed diet with very little sugar and yeast.

Summary

- Candida Albicans is a natural addition to our intestinal flora but it becomes overgrown when we adopt a highly processed diet, ingest certain prescribed medications such as anti-biotics, or we suffer from repeated stomach upsets.
- Yeast and Sugar are the food of choice for the Candida in your gut and to get the overgrowth under control you need to eliminate as many processed sources of that as possible.
- There are about 120 symptoms associated with a Candida Overgrowth, *one of which is a reduced sex drive and subsequent sexual dysfunction.*
- Following the Healthy Eating Plan for life at the back of the book will minimise the amount of sugars that you are including on a daily basis.
- Remember to check labels for sugar in any processed foods that you eat

Candida Questionnaire

You will note that there are questions regarding female reproduction in the list. I suggest that if you have a partner that they complete this questionnaire too, as you may find that if one of you suffers from Candida that you both might.

Score 0 if rare, 1 if often

Digestion	Score
Gas	
Intestinal pain	
Belching after most foods	
Constipation or Diarrhoea	
Chronic heartburn	
Haemorrhoids	
Dry mouth	
Bad breath	
Craving for sugars	
Craving for breads	
Craving for alcohol	
Total	

Drug Use	Score
Tetracycline: Used for less than 1 month: score 1 For longer use: score 2	
Cortisone: Less than 2 weeks: score 1 More than 2 weeks: score 2	

Drug Use	Score
Antibiotics: Used over a period of 2 months or longer, or more than 4 times in any one year: score 10 Any use of antibiotics: score 6	
Birth control pill More than 2 years: score 2 Less than 2 years: score 1	
Total	

Allergy	Score
Earache or constant discharge	
Hives	
Asthma	
Sensitivity to certain foods	
Mucus (body, nose, throat.)	
Wheezing	
Headaches	
Itching nose	
Rashes or allergic reactions	
Fungus infection between toes	
Burning or watering eyes, with discharge	
Total	

Nerves & Stress	Score
Headaches or Migraine	
Depression	
Persistent Tiredness	
Poor Concentration	
Panic attacks	
Low energy	
Dizziness or vertigo	
Insomnia	
Total	

Genito-urinary	Score
Yeast Infections (e.g. Thrush)	
Menstrual irregularities, cramping pains	
Cystitis	
Endometriosis	
Total	

Have you ever been pregnant?	Score
Once: score 3	
Two or more times: score 5	
Total	

Combined Score for all Questions	

How To Analyse Your Scores

1-5   Indicates that Candida is under control.

5-15   Normal, but Candida needs to be watched.
Use mild Candida diet and treat any irritating symptoms.

15-30   Indicates moderate Candida
Change to Candida diet and treat symptoms.

30+   Indicates severe Candida.
Seek advice from a qualified Nutritional Therapist

17. Acidity Can Be Contributory Factor in Poor Sex Drive

You have had a great night out – a couple of drinks and a large Indian meal and you are now in the mood. Except you have violent indigestion and suddenly your mind is elsewhere and sex is off the menu!

The word acid comes from the Latin word acere, which means sour. The term has been applied to chemical compounds containing the element hydrogen and having the ability to supply positively charged hydrogen ions to a chemical reaction.

Most acids are sour as opposed to most alkalis, which are bitter. Acid is also corrosive to metals and will change litmus (a dye from lichens) red and neutralise alkalines.

All acids have similar properties to each other because they all release hydrogen into solutions.

Acidity is measured using the pH (potential of hydrogen) scales. The scale runs from 0 to 14. All acids have a pH measurement between 0 to below 7 on the scale.

Acids are present in all living organisms including the human body. Acids in plants react differently than acids in protein rich foods such as animal products. All foods are burned in the body leaving an ash as a result, if the food contains a predominance of sulphur, phosphorus, chlorine then an acid ash is produced.

The body has developed different strategies to ensure that the balance between acid and alkali is optimum for each of its different organs and systemic functions.

For example citrus fruit, in particular one that has a sour taste like the lemon, contains high levels of citric acid and is classified as an acid food. However, the ash that is produced is alkaline. The negative charges on the citrate ions are balanced by positively charged metal ions, such as calcium and potassium. The citrate is oxidised away during this process to carbon dioxide and water and excreted leaving the calcium and potassium behind. As alkalis they in turn are balanced by other acidic properties such as bicarbonate or chloride to ensure that the correct pH balance is maintained. This is an alkaline reaction resulting from ingesting an acid food.

Most animal proteins contain sulphur amino acids and phosphoprotein. When these are metabolised by the body they become sulphuric and phosphoric acids. Therefore these foods are said to be acid forming.

The lower the pH level, the higher the acidity forming property of the food.

Optimum health and energy begins as with every function in our bodies with balance. The pH balance of our bodies is not only crucial, it is the essence of our survival and the body has evolved very efficient methods of maintaining this critical balance of acidity and alkalinity in our blood and the major organs of the body. All cells, organs and fluids have their own preferred pH values in order to operate at peak performance.

Outside influences as well as internal balancing strategies play a part in effecting the pH balance of the body. Stress, diet, nutrition, levels of exercise and environmental pollution are a major part of our lives today and most of our chronic illnesses are associated with our bodies becoming more acidic than alkaline.

A minor deviation from the optimum balance can have a devastating effect on the operating systems of the body and can lead to coma and death so the body has a number of buffer systems to maintain that balance. When the blood is too alkaline the heart contracts and ceases to beat and when too acidic it relaxes and ceases to beat.

One of the buffers the body uses to maintain the acid/alkali balance is the use of LDL (low density lipoprotein) which binds to acids from fluids such as blood or lymphatic systems. It enables the acid to be excreted safely from the body in urine.

Alkaline salts are also used to buffer acids. These are sodium, potassium, calcium and magnesium, which are held in reserve in bone and tissue. When there is excess acid produced, these salts are taken from the reserve to bind with the acids and neutralise them. The acids are then eliminated from the body through the colon, kidneys, lungs and skin. The strength of the survival instinct in the body is so strong that the balance of acid/alkaline will be maintained even if it means removal of these alkaline salts from other sources. If the reserves are not available this means that calcium for example is leeched from bone, leaving the body vulnerable to diseases such as osteoporosis.

When we exercise hard, lactic acid and carbon dioxide are produced. Carbon dioxide in fluid becomes carbonic acid, which is a volatile acid now dissolved in the bloodstream. This changes the pH of the blood making it more acidic. A reaction must therefore take place to return the blood pH levels to the safe level of 7.4. We breathe deeply and rapidly and the concentration of carbon dioxide in the alveoli of the lungs is lowered and the lungs then remove carbon dioxide from the blood. The carbonic acid (H2CO3) loses its CO2 leaving H2O or water. This returns the acidic level to normal.

If a person has a health problem they are most likely acidic. Unless the body's pH level is slightly alkaline it cannot heal itself. It will not matter what type of therapy you use to take care of a specific health problem, as it will not be effective until the pH level is up. Additionally, unless the body is within the correct range it will be unable to absorb or utilise efficiently any vitamins, minerals or other nutrients from the diet.

There are certain health problems that are more likely to be associated with an acid/alkaline imbalance, including Osteoporosis, Arthritis, Diabetes, High Blood pressure, ME, Candida Albicans, Kidney stones, Acid reflux and cancer among many.

Ideally you would test pH levels using pH paper. Urine and saliva are tested first thing in the morning and levels noted. The normal range for saliva is 6.8 to 7.4 and is normally alkaline. If the test result indicates that it is lower than 6.8 then there is acid present in the system. Urine although more acidic should be within the range of 6.4 to 6.8. Below this and it would indicate abnormal levels of acidity.

Without the test then symptoms would need to be investigated. Some of the early indications would be acne, muscular pain, cold hands and feet, low energy, food intolerances, bloating, heartburn, mild headaches and a metallic taste in the mouth. A more intense acidity in the system may have escalated these symptoms to Migraine headaches, constipation, cold sores, loss of concentration, disturbances to smell, taste or vision.

Other indications would be frequent bacterial, viral and fungal infections, urinary tract infections and skin problems.

Apart from determining the type of foods that might be contributing to high acidity such as excess animal proteins, high grain and low plant food diets, lifestyle and emotional stresses need to be considered.

The aim is to implement an eating plan that incorporates Alkaline forming foods and Acid forming foods in a ratio of 4-to-1 or 80% alkaline forming and 20% acid forming.

Exercises will be needed to help reduce stress levels and improve breathing techniques. The rate that a person breathes has a direct effect on the acid or alkaline balance. Breathing exercises will greatly reduce the level of acidity in the body and are easy to do once or twice a day. I look at stress a little further on in the book in more detail and in the exercise section of the book you will find breathing exercises that will help you relax.

To ensure maximum nutritional uptake from the alkaline foods that are being included in the diet the recommendation would be that at least 50% of the foods be eaten raw and unprocessed. Most green leaf vegetables, root vegetables such as carrot and fruits are all edible in a raw state and very nutritious. Particular foods to be included with a high alkaline ash residue would be all fruits and most vegetables including tomatoes, avocados, carrots, dried fruit, olives, shitake mushrooms, and orange juice. Proteins such as whole milk and buttermilk and whole grains such as millet can be included as well as neutral foods such as butter.

Foods to be avoided would include Rice bran and dried fish, fried foods, processed foods (high Phosphorus) and drinks such as sodas and caffeine. Other foods can be incorporated into the diet in the correct proportion such as eggs, fish, beef, lamb and whole grains. There are many benefits to brown rice as a whole grain for example, not only its nutritional content but also its properties in assisting the body to eliminate toxins and help lower cholesterol levels. The same with proteins such as salmon and chicken provided they only form 20% of the diet they can be included.

The body will need to be hydrated to assist in flushing out the toxins and maintaining the correct fluid balance in the cells and tissues.

Summary

- The alkaline and acid balance in our bodies is critical and needs to be maintained for good health.
- If you are suffering from acid indigestion then it is a good sign that you need to change some aspects of your diet.
- Every food also has an alkaline or acid value and surprisingly lemons which you might think of as being acid actually burn to an alkaline ash in the body which is why they are included in the healthy eating plan for life.
- Eating the majority of your fruit and vegetables raw is a way to reduce the acid reaction in the body.
- High acid foods include sugars, high fat meats and eating a very high grain diet.

18. Why Is Refined Sugar so Bad for Us?

In the last few chapters I have covered Diabetes, Candida Albicans overgrowth and Acidity. All of these contribute to obesity, disease and in the long run will contribute to sexual dysfunction. Knowing ones enemy is very important. If you are to eliminate something from your diet, particularly something which so many people are addicted to you have understand what it is and how it works.

Sugar in the Modern Diet

Before we look at sugar as food in its own right we need to first look at the food group that it belongs in.

Sugars are a form of carbohydrate, which is our main source of energy. Carbohydrates are a group of nutrients that contain carbon atoms that have been hydrated by adding water molecules, hence the name carbohydrates. Carbohydrates include sugars, starches and fibre. The sugars and starches are metabolised by the body into the simple sugar, glucose. Glucose molecules circulate in the bloodstream, supplying our cells with the fuel, as they need it. Any additional glucose is converted in to glycogen, which is stored in the muscles of the liver. If your storehouse is already full then any excess glucose gets converted into fat.

Are There Different Types of Carbohydrate?

There are two types of carbohydrate, simple and complex. Simple carbohydrates contain one or two saccharides such as sucrose (glucose and fructose) which is table sugar and lactose (glucose and galactose) which is the sugar found in milk. This is called a disaccharide.

If a carbohydrate only has one saccharide it is called monosaccharide such as fructose which is the sugar found in fruit and honey. The less saccharides the sweeter the taste and the sweetest sugar therefore is fructose.

Complex carbohydrates are known as polysaccharides and they are made of long strings of the simple sugars and there are many different kinds. These are the starches and are the most nutritious because they tend to be a component in a food that has other nutrients.

The body also breaks down starches into glucose but it takes longer to digest than the simple sugars so they don't cause the same blood sugar fluctuations.

Fibre is a very important carbohydrate because the body, in particular the intestine does not have the enzymes necessary to break down the long chain into individual sugars molecules so it does not get absorbed into the bloodstream. Instead as part of another complex carbohydrate it slows down the digestion and absorption of sugar, which extends and maintains the energy levels provided.

Why Is Consuming Too Much Simple Carbohydrate in the Form of Sugars Bad for You?

Again I am not suggesting that you exclude sugars from your life altogether but certainly reducing the amount you consume will have a positive effect not only on your weight but on most of your bodies necessary functions. Here are some of the harmful effects of too much sugar in your diet. The list is really quite extensive and I am only including a handful but it does give you an idea of the short and long-term damage that is likely.

Eating too much sugar in your diet can suppress your immune system, cause behavioural problems in children, cause kidney damage, and increase levels of LDL (lousy cholesterol) and the even more damaging decrease in levels of HDL (healthy cholesterol).

It can cause nutrient deficiencies such as chromium (stable blood sugar levels) copper, calcium and magnesium.

It has been linked to diseases such as Candida, cancer, diabetes, heart disease, varicose veins, high blood pressure, eye disease, depression and liver and kidney problems. There are many other conditions that are worsened by obesity, which is often linked to high intakes of simple carbohydrates in the form of sugars as well as fats. All of the above of course are also causes of sexual dysfunction and it makes sense to address this one thing in your diet above all else to reduce your risk of some serious and chronic diseases.

One of the Biggest Medical Concerns Is the Increase in Levels of Diabetes 2 – What Is the Link to Sugar Consumption?

Refined sugars in table sugar and in most processed foods such as chocolate; biscuits and cakes are called rapid sugars. They do not need to be digested and are absorbed almost immediately into our bloodstream. In excessive amounts they raise the level of our blood glucose and this is called hyperglycaemia. The pancreas releases insulin to counteract this rise in blood glucose but it is difficult for a balance to be achieved if the intake of sugar is continuous, which results in too much insulin reducing the blood glucose level too low resulting in hypoglycaemia. Symptoms of this would be depression, dizziness, insomnia, weakness and in extreme cases unconsciousness.

Another effect of the blood glucose falling too low is the stress on the adrenal glands, which have to mobilise the stores of glycogen in the liver and our muscle to act as a referee between sugar and insulin. The adrenal glands and the pancreas are now both weakened which leads for an isolated incidence of hypoglycaemia to full blown diabetes.

Does a Heavy Intake of Sugars Affect Any of Our Other Glands and Functions?

Sometimes you will hear people talk about a sugar rush and how they cannot go a day without eating chocolate or having sugar in their tea or coffee. Part of this is because sugar stimulates a stress reaction, which increases our production of adrenaline (fight or flight hormone) by four times the normal amount. This in turn increases the production of cortisone, which inhibits immune system function.

Sugars do not have the nutrients themselves to metabolise so they have to take these out of our stores. If you have a high intake of sugar and are continually depleting your nutritional reserves without putting much back you will lower the effectiveness of your defences.

If We Have a Sweet Tooth, How Can We Reduce Our Intake?

Do remember that it is your taste buds that have the craving not necessarily you. Although you may need the high that a sugar fix gives you, the intensity of the sweetness is determined on the tongue. Like salt, after a few days you will begin to notice that you are finding certain foods too sweet and will take in less.

Drinking lots of sodas does nothing to help you. Move to drinking fresh squeezed fruit juices and water. In the healthy eating plan it is recommended that you cut down alcohol intake, as this is primarily sugars and again you will find that this will help with sugar cravings.

If you are a heavy meat eater you will find there is a corresponding requirement for sugars. In the first week of reducing your sugar intake, switch to fish for the week, particularly salmon and the other fatty fishes as this will help.

Use chopped fruit on your cereal or a handful of raisins. Mash a banana on buttered toast rather than use jam or marmalade.

Reduce your intake over a period of weeks. Going cold turkey if you can is great but it is less stressful and more likely to work if you give up your daily chocolate, biscuits and pastry to every other day and then to perhaps once or twice a week.

Look at food labels and check out how much carbohydrate – of which sugars etc. is on the packet. Compare labels and go for the packet that has the least sugar. Do remember that you are also looking for the alternative sugars and you should try and avoid these wherever possible.

Soft Drinks

There is little doubt that drinking too much alcohol is bad for your health in many respects. Your liver, brain and immune system come under immense pressure when they have to deal with excessive amounts and the long term affect on health is measurable. However, these days, the alternatives that are on every shelf of the supermarket and in bars and restaurants should not be the first thing you turn to when moderating your alcohol consumption.

The worst offenders are the carbonated drinks. Fruit juices without added sugars and additives mixed with mineral water or undiluted are fine in moderation. They too are high in fruit acids that can cause some tooth damage if you do not clean your teeth at least twice a day, particularly at night. It is the processed canned and bottled fizzy drinks that really do have some harmful effects on not only the teeth but also our operational systems in the body and structural health of skin and bones.

Does the Acid in Coke Have a Specific Effect on Any Part of the Body?

When you introduce the acid in Coke or Pepsi to your stomach acid it immediately increases the levels of acid dramatically. It causes an inflammation of the stomach and erosion of the stomach lining, which results in very severe stomach aches. Part of the problem is the combination of caffeine and acids in soft drinks, which include acetic, fumaric, gluconic and phosphoric acids.

The stomach maintains a very delicate acid/alkaline balance to enable your food to be digested and then metabolised efficiently. You can see now that by just having one or two soft drinks that this balance is disrupted but in the quantities that most people drink them, there is the distinct possibility of severe damage.

Eventually with constant increased acidity levels there will be erosion of the gastric lining, the phosphorous which is found in high levels in soft drinks will effectively neutralise the hydrochloric acid in the stomach acid, making the digestive process ineffective and this results in bloating and gas.

Carbon dioxide is produced when we consume the soft drink and this depletes the amount of oxygen in the body and some researchers are beginning to connect to this to increased risks to cancer from damaged cells.

What About the Caffeine That Is in Some Soft Drinks?

Caffeine is a mild drug; in adults too much can elevate blood pressure and cause anxiety. In young children it can cause hyperactivity as it acts a stimulant on the nervous system and they can also suffer from insomnia, anxiety, irritability and irregular heart beats. Caffeine is addictive and this causes the drinker to want more and more of the soft drinks. It is not unusual for people to drink one can after another much like a chain smoker and cigarettes.

Is There Anything Else That Causes Concern in Soft Drinks?

Apart from the preservatives and additives we have already talked about there are the colouring agents that are used. In particular your lovely dark, bubbly glass of cola did not originally start out as brown in colour. That is due to the caramel colouring caused by the chemical polyethylene glycol which is antifreeze – there are concerns that this is carcinogenic.

Summary

We tend to put food in our mouths without really putting a nutritional value on it or considering its harmful affects. This is particularly so with sugars which tend to be hidden in much of the food that we eat. Even if we think we are eating healthily we rarely quantify the ingredients we are consuming. How many times have you prepared an Italian dish, for example, and used a jar of pasta sauce assuming that the meal was savoury and sugar free. Next time you are in the supermarket check the amount of carbohydrates on the label and then look and see how much of that is sugars. Do the same with your bowl of breakfast cereal especially if it is honey coated (not really honey).

- You should have no more than 10 level teaspoons of sugar each day.
- You need to have a conversion figure for sugar included on the label. 4 gm of sugar equals 1 teaspoon of sugar.
- If the label states that there is 40 gm of sugar per serving then you will be consuming 10 teaspoons of sugar or your entire daily allowance in one go.
- Additionally, 1 gm of sugar is 4 calories which means that you will also have consumed 160 calories in that serving. These are what we refer to as hidden sugars but they are also hidden calories too.

19. Stress and Sexual Performance

If you are reading this book because you would like to improve your sex life then you will already be aware that when you are under stress there is more likelihood that you are unable to enjoy sex either physically or emotionally. If you have had a dreadful day at the office – experiencing financial difficulties – have relationship problems it is not going to make you feel inclined to relax and enjoy the moment.

Today stress plays an enormous part in all our lives, men, women and children are affected in one way or another. Stress is actually an important reaction to an event or events that might threaten us. It is also part of the adrenaline rush that you feel when you are in the middle of performing something that is perhaps outside your comfort zone. Managing stress however, can be the tricky bit as too much can cause many physical health problems one being of course sexual dysfunction.

What Is Stress?

There are two types of stress, Acute Stress and Chronic Stress, and both have very distinctive patterns.

Acute Stress is a short-term response by the body's sympathetic nervous system and the response may only last for a few minutes or a few weeks. How many times have you said that your heart stopped or your stomach lurched during a moment of intense stress such as an accident? We have all heard stories of mothers and fathers who have been suddenly infused with superhuman strength and able to lift cars and other heavy objects off their trapped children. They are empowered to do this by the actions of their body in a moment of crisis.

Blood sugar levels rise and additional red blood cells are released to carry strength giving oxygen levels a boost. The pulse quickens, blood pressure rises and the digestive process stops to enable the focus to be entirely on regaining safety.

Chronic Stress is when this acute stress response is repeated on a continuous basis. Whilst the body, after a hundred thousand years, is well able to handle the occasional stress response and in fact uses it positively, if the response becomes a normal way of life, other parts of the brain and body become involved leading to long term damage.

For example, ongoing stress causes the hypothalamus and the pituitary gland, which are the master controllers for the body, to release a chemical called ACTH (adrenocorticotropic hormone) which stimulates the adrenal gland to produce and release cortisol which disrupts sleep patterns leading to increased levels of stress. Our bodies are simply not designed to live at high alert for sustained periods of time; it just wears it down leading to illness.

Firstly though some basic techniques to help you manage whatever stress you do have in your lives. It would be a perfect world where we had absolutely no worries whatsoever but I am afraid there are only a few people who live in that serene an environment.

It is easier said than done, but you must find a way to relax that suits you. Think carefully about what makes you feel alive but calm, that gives you satisfaction and creates a feel good factor. For you as an individual it could be skiing down a mountain or it could be walking along a sandy beach at sunset. As unique as the causes of stress are so are the ways that we find to counteract the tension. It might be that you have several physical, mental and emotional activities that you find distracting and calming. A game of tennis, followed by doing the Sunday crossword and then watching a weepy movie. Certainly you will find it very beneficial to learn some deep breathing techniques. Counting to ten before blowing your top can actually be very effective.

If you really cannot think of anything on your own then find yourself a professional advisor who can help you find your bit of space and peace. It is always a good idea to find someone who has been referred by a friend or family member but your GP should also be able to recommend someone.

Keep to a regular sleep pattern, although people do need varying amounts of sleep the average is seven hours. Go to bed at the same time each night and get up at the same time even at the weekends.

Lack of sleep is one of the leading causes of stress. After several nights of less than your normal quota you will begin to feel stressed and also very tired.

I am afraid that stimulants such as cigarettes and alcohol and recreational drugs are absolutely the wrong things to rely on during a stress episode, as hard as it may be, avoid these at all costs.

Diet and Stress

A healthy diet is absolutely necessary whatever lifestyle we have but if we are under excessive levels of stress then it becomes critical.

Make sure that you are hydrated. Dehydration is a leading physical cause of stress and you need at least 2 litres of fresh, pure water per day and more if you are on holiday or living in very hot climates.

Seven Good Reasons to Drink Water

1. Your body consists of between 60% and 75% water.
2. Each day our body loses 2 litres of fluid through urination, Breathing and through our skin. We require even more fluids in warm climates or if we have a higher activity level.
3. Not drinking enough fluids puts a great deal of stress on the body. Kidney function particularly will be affected and there is a danger of kidney and gallstones forming. Immune function is impaired leaving us more prone to infection.
4. Lack of water causes a number of problems that we tend to shrug off. Headaches, irritability (especially first thing in the morning and in children) aching legs, water retention, poor skin tone, circles under the eyes, dull and lifeless hair, lack of energy and poor emulsification of fats.
5. Drinking water helps prevent water retention. Your body knows that it will die very rapidly without fluids so it tends to keep as much as it can in reserve.
6. If you are taking regular medication basis you need to make sure that you flush your system daily to ensure that there is no build up of toxins in your cells, kidneys and liver.
7. There are some vitamins and minerals which the body needs to handle stress especially as during a stress interval the body will use up additional reserves of many nutrients. Lots of fresh fruit and vegetables are necessary and here

are a few of the particular nutrients that will help you handle the stress in your life. In the section of the book on the nutrients we need to be healthy on a daily basis I will go into each of these in more detail but this is a snapshot to get you started.

Stress Vitamins

- Vitamin A mops up the toxic residue of elevated stress hormone levels. (Liver, fish oils, butter, cheese, Free range eggs, oily fish and Beta-carotene that converts to Vitamin A from carrots, green leafy vegetables such as asparagus and broccoli, orange and red coloured vegetables such as apricots)
- Vitamin B1 improves your mood and is vital for nerve function. (Whole grains, seeds, peas, beans and nuts.)
- Vitamin B3 helps you regulate your sleep patterns. (Liver, brewer's yeast, chicken, turkey, fish, meat, peanuts, whole-grains, eggs and milk.)
- Vitamin B5, better known as Pantothenic Acid, controls the action of the adrenal glands, which play a vital part in the stress response. (Liver, yeast, salmon, dairy, eggs, grains, meat and vegetables.)
- Vitamin B6 is essential for the manufacture of the brain chemical serotonin, which is also called the feel good chemical. (Potatoes, bananas, cereals, lentils, liver, turkey, chicken, lamb, fish, avocados, soybeans, walnuts and oats.)
- Vitamin B12 is necessary to help produce brain chemicals such as serotonin (dairy, eggs, meat, poultry and fish, for vegetarians in Miso and Tempeh both fermented soybean products)
- Vitamin C is one of those vitamins that is used up very quickly during a stress reaction and needs to be replaced immediately as a deficiency leads to increased levels of anxiety and irritability. Smokers should take in Vitamin C in their diet and under the supervision of a professional should also take supplemental Vitamin C. (found in all fruit and vegetables but best sources are blackcurrants, broccoli, Brussels sprouts, cabbage, cauliflower, cherries, grapefruits, guavas, kiwi fruit, lemons, parsley, peppers, rosehips, potatoes, tomatoes and watercress.)

Minerals Essential To Help the Body Manage Stress

Calcium helps you relax and studies have certainly shown that for women it can help reduce the symptoms of stress related to their periods. (Dairy, sardines, canned salmon with the bones, green leafy vegetables such as spinach and soy products such as tofu.)

Magnesium works with calcium and also helps to reduce stress. (Whole grains, beans, seeds, wheat germ, dried apricots, dark green vegetables, soybeans and fish)

Chromium stabilises blood sugar levels that create stress. (Brewer's yeast, onions, whole grains, shellfish, liver and molasses)

The aim of a healthy diet is to provide your body with the necessary fuel in the right proportions to enable it to achieve homeostasis, or balance. If you are living a very stressful lifestyle then you need to ensure that you address that balance as quickly as possible. If you suffer from low to moderate levels of stress you will find that by adopting relaxation techniques and giving your body the correct fuel to deal with the situation will have long lasting and very beneficial effects on you now and also years ahead in the future. Don't allow your stress levels today creep up on you unawares in 20 years time, deal with it today.

Part Two –
Essential Nutrients, Vitamins & Minerals

Getting the Right Fuel Mix!

In Part One I gave you a brief overview of the lifestyle conditions that can lead to sexual dysfunction as well as general ill health.

I hope that you can now see that there are usually a combination of factors that lead to any chronic disease and body malfunction and that you can have a hand in not only repairing the damage but returning to a higher quality of health and life.

I often use the car as an analogy for my clients because it has many working parts, requires a cocktail of chemicals to make it fire on all cylinders and ceases to move when it is not given the correct fuel mix. For example if you drive a non-leaded petrol vehicle you will not be doing the engine any favours by putting diesel into it.

Unfortunately most of us go through life with an unleaded engine battling to function on not only diesel fuel but fuel that is full of contaminants. Additives, preservatives and colourants in the processed food that makes up a high percentage of our diet form an unholy alliance in our system which strives to survive and function. We end up with systems that may only have 50% efficiency and we then wonder why we suffer frequent infections, have no energy or lose our sex drive. When the body is under pressure and is not getting the nutrients it requires to be healthy it will sacrifice the unnecessary functions in favour of survival.

Your body is also like a factory which has a number of processes running in parallel to provide the final product. If you interrupt the conveyor belt at any stage the finished product is going to be missing parts. Usually the body will affect a work around but as we all know these are rarely permanent or successful.

You could skip this part of course and head straight to the eating plan at the back of the book. However, wouldn't you like to know some of the ingredients that are critically necessary to make the fuel you put into your bodies high octane? Without these nutrients you will not fire on all cylinders and you will not be giving your body the chance to enjoy the sex life that you desire.

I used to think that talking about vitamins and minerals was boring and unproductive but as I learnt more about the human body and its amazing abilities to survive my efforts at self destruction, I came to respect and appreciate their value.

I am not writing a compendium of nutrients but I would like to give you the fundamentals of the nutrients we need to live and be healthy. In the following section you then find the foods that I consider to be packed with these nutrients and should be included in your diet on a regular basis.

Our individual biochemical makeup will determine our health throughout our lifetime. Everyday life in this modern world puts stress on our bodies and with an inadequate diet, our bodies are unable to maintain health and well being and we can develop diseases that harm and age us. Our bodies have used food as a fuel and to sustain our health throughout our evolution. There is an abundance of nutrient packed food right on our doorstep and if we follow a largely fresh, unprocessed diet we can obtain the majority of the nutrients we require for good health and long life. In certain circumstances then it may be advisable to take additional nutrients in the form of supplements, but always the first place to start is ensuring that you are taking in the maximum amount of nutrients through food sources.

I have listed the main nutrients that we require every day. The list is not exhaustive but is designed to show you just how much nutrition you can obtain from a healthy diet of readily available food.

Whilst you might like to skip the next section and go straight to the healthy eating plan I would like you to bear in mind that knowing what the components are of your optimum fuel mix will enable you to keep your motor running for several hundred thousand miles!

Something for Your Hormones

Essential Fatty Acids (EFAs)

Essential Fatty Acids (EFAs) are necessary fats that humans cannot synthesise and must be obtained through diet. There are two families of EFAs Omega-3 and Omega-6. Omega-9 is necessary but non-essential as the body can make it if the other two fatty acids are present.

EFAs are essential because they support our cardiovascular, reproductive, immune and nervous systems. We need these fats to manufacture and repair cells, maintain hormone levels and expel waste from the body. They are part of the process that regulates blood pressure, blood clotting, fertility and conception – and they also help regulate inflammation and stimulate the body to fight infection.

Omega-3 (Linolenic Acid) is the principal Omega-3 fatty acid and is used in the formation of cell walls, improving circulation and oxygen. A deficiency can lead to decreased immune system function; elevated levels of LDL (bad cholesterol) high blood pressure and irregular heart beat. It is also anti-inflammatory and helps prevent heart disease. It is found in flaxseed, walnuts, pumpkinseeds, avocados, spinach and other dark green leafy vegetables, sardines, tuna and salmon.

Omega-6 (Linoleic Acid) is the primary Omega-6 fatty acid. Omega-6 can improve rheumatoid arthritis, lower blood cholesterol, PMS, skin problems such as eczema and psoriasis. Found in flaxseeds, pumpkinseeds, olive oil, evening primrose oil, chicken and poultry, salmon.

There is growing evidence that the non-essential Oleic acid, Omega-9, may help to lower cholesterol by decreasing the unhealthy cholesterol, LDL (low-density lipoprotein), while at the same time raising the level of healthy cholesterol, HDL (high density lipoprotein).

Oleic acid is also emerging as a regulator of blood-sugar levels and as a possible protection against breast and prostate cancer. So, including half an avocado in your diet every day may well protect you from the harmful long-term affects of a number of diseases. Found in olive oil, olives, avocados, almonds, and walnuts.

A Closer Look at Why EFAs are so Essential.

First and foremost EFAs provide us with energy but unlike saturated fats their effect is beneficial. The body cannot manufacture them and that is why it is ESSENTIAL to include them on a daily basis in your diet.

Both of the important EFA families – omega-6 and omega-3 – are components of nerve cells and cellular membranes. They are converted by the body into hormone like messengers such as prostaglandins – which are needed on a second-by-second basis by most tissue activities in the body.

EFAs are involved in:
- Regulating pressure in the eye, joints, and blood vessels.
- dilating or constricting blood vessels
- directing endocrine hormones to specific cells
- regulating smooth muscle reflexes
- being the main constituent of cell membranes
- regulating the rate of cell division
- regulating the inflow and outflow of substances to and from cells
- transporting oxygen from red blood cells to the tissues
- maintaining proper kidney function and fluid balance
- keeping saturated fats mobile in the bloodstream
- preventing blood cells from clumping together (blood clots that can be a cause of heart attack and stroke)
- minimising the release of inflammatory substances from cells that may trigger allergic conditions
- regulating nerve transmission and communication
- If the diet is deficient in either omega-6 or omega-3 long-term degenerative illnesses can result such as arthritis, Alzheimer's disease and heart disease.

Amino Acids

There are two types of amino acid, essential and non-essential. There are approximately 80 amino acids found in nature but only

20 are necessary for healthy human growth and function. We are made up of protein and we require adequate amounts of amino acids if we are to maintain and repair the very substance that we are made from.

We need to obtain essential amino acids from our diet and our body will produce the nonessential variety on its own if our diet is lacking in the essential type.

Essential Amino Acids

These are Histidine (essential in infants can be made by the body in adults if needed), Isoleucine, Leucine, Lysine, Methionine, Cysteine (essential in infants, nonessential in adults), Phenylalanine, Threonine, Tryptophan and Valine.

Nonessential Amino Acids

Alanine, Aspartic acid, Arginine, Carnitine, Glycine, Glutamine, Hydroxyglumatic acid, Hydroxyproline, Norleucine, Proline, Serine and Tyrosine.

The Role of Amino Acids in the Body

Amino acids help make neurotransmitters, the chemicals that convey messages in the brain and also hormones like insulin. They are needed for the production of enzymes that activate certain functions within the body and certain types of body fluid and they are essential for the repair and maintenance of organs, glands, muscles, tendons, ligaments, skin, hair and nails.

An Example of One of the Amino Acids

Tryptophan is an excellent example of the role of amino acids within the body.

When we eat foods that contain tryptophan the body will use that to form the very important vitamin B3 or Niacin. Niacin is necessary for the metabolism of carbohydrates, fats and proteins to obtain the fuel we need (ATP) as well as helping to regulate cholesterol. It is necessary for the formation of red blood cells and hormones including the sex hormones.

When niacin is formed it continues to work with the tryptophan along with B6 to stimulate the production of the serotonin and melatonin transmitters within the brain that not only help regulate our mood but also our sleep patterns. Without tryptophan we would be more likely to suffer from insomnia and depression.

Cysteine plays a role in our antioxidant processes protecting us from free radical damage and therefore chronic disease and ageing. It is currently being studied in relation to a number of medical conditions including peptic ulcers, liver health, the treatment of paracetamol overdose and metal toxicity.

It may also benefit respiratory disease due to its antioxidant properties but also its ability to help break up mucous. In the form of N-acetyl cysteine it may protect the body from cancer and there is a possibility that during treatment for cancer with chemotherapy or radiotherapy that it will protect the healthy cells but not the cancerous cells from any damage.

When we looked at heart disease we covered the role of homocysteine levels in the blood and how excess levels can lead to heart disease. Taking N-acetyl cysteine in supplement form may help reduce these levels as well as the LDL (lousy cholesterol levels) in the blood.

Brief Description of Some of the Other Amino Acids and Their Role in the Body

There is not room to cover the roles within the body of all the amino acids but here is a brief look at the diverse roles of some of the individual amino acids within the body.

ALANINE

A very simple amino acid involved in the energy producing breakdown of glucose and is used to build proteins, vital for the function of the central nervous system and helps form neurotransmitters. It is very important to promote proper blood glucose levels derived from dietary protein.

ARGININE

Plays an important role in healthy cell division, wound healing, removing ammonia from the body, boosting the immune system and in the production and release of hormones.

CARNITINE

Is produced in the liver, brain and kidneys from the essential amino acids methionine and lysine. It is the nutrient responsible for the transport of fatty acids into the energy producing centres of the cells, known as the mitochondria. It also helps promote healthy heart muscle.

CYSTEINE

Plays a role in our antioxidant processes protecting us from free radical damage and therefore chronic disease and ageing. It is currently being studied in relation to a number of medical conditions including peptic ulcers, liver health, the treatment of paracetamol overdose and metal toxicity.

CREATINE

Is synthesised in the liver, kidneys and pancreas from Arginine, Methionine and Glycine and functions to increase the availability of the fuel we need ATP (adenosine triphosphate). It is stored in muscle cells and is used to generate cellular energy for muscle contractions when effort is required. This is why many athletes will supplement with Creatine to increase stamina and performance.

Food Sources for Amino Acids

The best food sources of amino acids are dairy products, fish, meat, soybeans, nuts and seeds.

The Antioxidant

Although I am going to cover the main vitamins and mineral in more detail it is important to look at one group of nutrients within this category that work tirelessly on our behalf to keep our system clear of rust.

A free radical is a molecule. A normal molecule has an even number of electrons and is considered stable. Free radicals on the other hand have an uneven number of electrons and are unstable. They are desperate to be like the normal molecules so they have to steal from them to get another electron. This of course means that they have created another free radical. More and more cells become damaged and leave the body open to most diseases from cardiovascular to cancer.

The free-radicals cause cells to oxidise and die. The major damage is done to our DNA, which results in mutations and death of the cells. Our body does produce anti-oxidants and enzymes that can repair this damage if we eat healthily. However, as we get older so do our cells and it becomes harder to repair them and they die. This is ageing! In our brains when cells are damaged beyond repair you are susceptible to loss of co-ordination and memory and in extreme cases dementia.

To prevent this we need a diet that is very high in anti-oxidants, which work through the body immobilising free radicals and preventing damage. Cranberries contain one of the highest levels of anti-oxidants of most fruit and vegetables and that is why drinking at least one glass per day can help provide you with enough of these defensive players to protect your brain

Bioflavanoids

For those of us who enjoy chocolate or red wine it is a useful justification to insist we are getting the benefit of flavanoids. It is true that one square of 80% cocoa chocolate does contain some health benefits as does the relaxing affect of the occasional glass of red wine but more is not necessarily better! Trouble is there are other side effects to eating chocolate and drinking too much alcohol that can negate the benefits.

However, there is no doubt the bioflavonoids found within different categories of fresh foods can be beneficial to the body.

Bioflavonoids are polyphenolic compounds with very strong antioxidant properties that can help protect the body's cells from damage. This is why they have been linked in research to the improvement and maintenance of brain function in the elderly and the protection affect in reducing risk factors for developing chronic diseases such as arthritis and heart disease.

If you like they offer an antioxidant boost that backs up the basic nutrients that provide this benefit to the body and because they are found in such a wide variety of foods they are readily available in a healthy balanced diet rich in fruit, vegetables, tea and coffee.

As you look through the various foods that I have used to illustrate how high nutritional content can be you will see that there are a number of different flavanoids on offer which include

- Catechins – found in tea, chocolate and red wine
- Flavanoids – including Quercitin found in apples and onions
- Flavones – found in celery and citrus
- Anthocyanins which are a group that includes cyanidin malvidin and petunidin – found in the violet and red pigments found in fruit and vegetables
- Isoflavones – found in soy products

Whilst it is not important that you know all the different names for flavanoids it is important that you understand how powerful a simple apple or orange can be in the battle to protect your body. It is important to understand that as complex as our own bodies are, each natural unprocessed food you place in your mouth is a complex entity of its own.

You will never look at a piece of fruit or a serving of vegetables in quite the same way again.

Vitamins

Vitamin A: Retinol and Beta-Carotene

Vitamin A is essential for our healthy eyesight, especially at night. It helps the cells reproduce normally. It is also necessary for the health of our skin, the mucus membranes in our respiratory system, digestive and urinary tracts. Our bones and our soft tissues require Vitamin A as part of the complex nutrient cocktail that keeps them from disease.

For younger people, Vitamin A has a direct influence on their reproductive capabilities. It has been shown to have an effect on the function and development of sperm, ovaries and the placenta. The growth and normal development of the embryo and then the foetus depends on a good level of the vitamin in the diet.

Our immune system also requires a cocktail of anti-oxidants and nutrients to be robust enough to cope with the stress of modern life and disease. Vitamin A is vital for this healthy protection system.

It is a fat-soluble vitamin mainly found in meat in oils. The most abundant source is found in liver, fish liver oils, butter, cheese, free range eggs and oily fish.

Beta carotene is a substance from plants that the body converts to Vitamin A and the best sources are carrots, green leafy vegetables, orange and red coloured vegetables, apricots, asparagus, broccoli, cantaloupe melon, cashews, nectarines, peaches, peppers and spinach.

Vitamin B1: Thiamine

Vitamin B1 (Thiamin) is a water-soluble vitamin. This means that this, along with the other B vitamins and Vitamin C, travel through the bloodstream and any excess is eliminated in our urine. The body cannot store Thiamine but it is found in tissues within the body such as in the liver, heart, kidneys and the nervous system where it binds to enzymes. This does mean that these types of vitamins need to be replaced from our food continuously.

Thiamine helps fuel our bodies by converting blood sugar into energy. Every cell in the body requires it to form the fuel we run on called adenosine triphosphate (ATP). It also keeps our mucus membranes healthy and with other B vitamins is essential for a healthy nervous and cardiovascular system as well as muscular function.

It is very rare in this day and age in the Western world to find a person who is deficient in Thiamin. A lack of it can cause a disease called beriberi with symptoms of rapid heartbeat, muscle wasting, nerve problems and confusion. There have been babies who have suffered from this due to a lack of the vitamin in their formula and people who drink excessive amounts of alcohol can also develop beriberi.

Most commonly it is found in elderly people who have general malabsorption problems or a restricted diet. Some children with congenital heart disease may suffer a deficiency, as can patients undergoing kidney dialysis who should be prescribed B1 by their doctor.

As a supplement it is usually taken as part of a B-complex formulation and does work better with vitamin B2 and B3.

The best food sources are all whole grains such as brown rice and whole wheat, sunflower seeds, sesame seeds, pineapple, watermelon, spinach, oats, lentils, beans, peanuts, eggs, lean ham and pork.

Vitamin B2: Riboflavin

Like the other B vitamins, B2 plays an important role in energy production by ensuring the efficient metabolism of the food that we eat in the form of carbohydrates, fats and proteins. It plays a key role in our nutritional processes such as its help in processing amino acids. Amino acids are the building blocks of protein, which is the substance that we are made of. Twenty amino acids are needed to build the various different proteins used in the growth, repair and maintenance of our body tissues and whilst eleven of these are made by the body itself, the others must be obtained from our diet and processed by other agents including B2.

Vitamin B2 is a vitamin that is essential for metabolising carbohydrates to produce ATP (adenosine triphosphate) without which we would be totally lacking in energy. It also works with enzymes in the liver to eliminate toxins, which helps keep us clear of infection.

B2 is needed to change B6 and Folic Acid into an active and usable form so that our nervous system is protected. Folic acid is essential for healthy cell division and is needed before and during the first twelve weeks of pregnancy to help prevent birth defects. B2 is also part of the process that changes tryptophan, so important to our mental wellbeing, into niacin.

It is also needed for red blood cell formation, breathing, antibody protection and regulating human growth and reproduction. Without B2 we would not enjoy healthy skin, nails and hair. Our thyroid function can be compromised if we do not take in sufficient B2.

B2 works in conjunction with B1, B3 and B6 and as a supplement is more usually taken as part of a B complex. Incidences of deficiency are low but are more prevalent in alcoholics and have been found in people suffering from cataracts or sickle cell anaemia. It is more likely to be a problem in developing countries where there has been some link to preeclampsia in pregnant women.

Sufferers of chronic fatigue syndrome, whose chief symptom is lack of energy are often deficient in the B vitamins and again B2 would be included as part of a B-complex supplement.

Other areas where eating foods rich in B2 may be helpful are with migraines, headaches, cataracts, rheumatoid arthritis and also skin conditions such as anaemia and acne.

The vitamin is water-soluble and cannot be stored in the body except in very small amounts so needs to be replenished from diet every day.

Best food sources are Kidney, Liver, Fish, Milk, Wheat germ, Broccoli and all green leafy vegetables.

Vegetarians and Vegans must make sure that they are taking in all the B vitamins and eating a diet high in raw dark green vegetables like spinach and broccoli will help increase the amount available as cooking does destroy much of the nutrient content.

Vitamin B3: Niacin

Vitamin B3 is also known in different forms as Niacin, Nicotinic Acid, Nicotinamide and Nicinamide. When the vitamin was first discovered it was called nicotinic acid but there was a concern that it would be associated with nicotine in cigarettes, leading to the false assumption that somehow smoking might provide you with nutrients. It was decided to call it Niacin instead.

It works with other nutrients, particularly B1, B2, B5, B6 and biotin to break the carbohydrates, fats, and proteins in food down into energy. B3 itself is essential in this process and it goes further by aiding in the production of hydrochloric acid in the stomach to aid the digestion of food. It is actually involved in over 40 metabolic functions which show how important it is in our levels of energy on a daily basis.

We are at the mercy of toxins and harmful chemicals in the body that need to be eliminated efficiently to prevent build up and illness. B3 works with the body and other nutrients to achieve this. Additionally when we are under attack from bacteria and viruses that we have not managed to eliminate fast enough, B3 will also assist in the antioxidant processes within the body to help us heal faster.

Enzymes are unique substances that speed up chemical reactions in the body. They are necessary to produce the energy we need, the breakdown of dietary fats, and the production of certain hormones and cholesterol. In addition they are needed for the processing of genetic material (DNA) and the growth and healthy maturing of cells. B3 is essential for the efficiency of many of these enzymes.

One of the areas that B3 is used therapeutically is in the lowering of cholesterol. B3 actually lowers LDL (lousy cholesterol) and raises HDL (healthy cholesterol). In tests, supplemented B3 proved more effective than many of the normal cholesterol lowering drugs although there have been instances of side effects in the form of excessive flushing. High dosage of any vitamin therapy should only be undertaken with the supervision of a medical professional and there are a number of different forms of B3 supplementation that can be used to minimise side effects whilst still acting to reduce LDL and raise HDL.

Niacin improves circulation by relaxing arteries and veins. This benefits sufferers of Reynaud's disease and other circulatory problems such as varicose veins. In Reynaud's the worst symptom is the numbness and pain in the hands and feet in cold weather. Niacin increases blood flow to them reducing the symptoms. People who suffer from muscle cramps may also be obtaining too little B3.

It is rare in the Western world for anyone to be deficient in

Niacin. But, since B3 in its various forms has been shown to help improve symptoms of some of our most common ailments it does pose the question as to whether we are actually obtaining sufficient of the vitamin from our diet or not. If we do, are our digestive systems not working efficiently enough to process and utilise it?

Normally the body manages to absorb enough niacin from our daily diet to accomplish its tasks. Apart from digestion it is needed to keep the skin and nerves healthy and to help stabilise blood sugar levels. The body can also convert niacin from tryptophan the amino acid found in eggs, milk, poultry and fish which means that there is a wide range of foods available to us that provide the vitamin. It reacts with tryptophan to form serotonin and melatonin in the brain, both of which effect our moods and general feeling of well being.

B3 has also been shown to relieve acne, reduce migraines, IBS symptoms, gout, menstrual problems, multiple sclerosis, Osteoarthritis, vertigo, memory loss and gastric problems.

For those of us interested in maintaining our brain health and avoiding dementia conditions such as Alzheimer's disease, B3 could be an important ally as we get older.

Deficiency symptoms are general weakness or muscle weakness, depressed appetite, skin infections and digestive problems.

B3 is water soluble and therefore needs to be replenished daily from your diet it is found in liver, chicken, Turkey, salmon, swordfish, tuna, venison, eggs, cheese and milk. Plant sources include green leafy vegetables such as Asparagus, broccoli, carrots, dates, mushrooms, peanuts, potatoes, tomatoes, spinach, sunflower seeds and whole grains.

If you are suffering from Reynaud's disease, arthritis elevated cholesterol levels or depression you may find that taking a B-complex supplement of help. There is sufficient B3 in most quality supplements to augment the dietary B3. Brewer's yeast is a good source of all the B vitamins you can take in tablet form.

Vitamin B5: Pantothenic Acid

Vitamin B5, Pantothenic acid, gets its name from the Greek word pantos, meaning everywhere because it is available in such a wide variety of foods. The problem is that much of a foods B5 is lost through cooking, which in another reason for eating as many fruits and vegetables as possible in the raw state.

B5 is one of the eight water-soluble B vitamins which cannot be stored by the body and have to be replenished in your daily diet. We have already covered B1, B2, and B3 and B5 like the others plays an important role in the conversion of carbohydrates into glucose, which is burned to produce energy. They are also needed to breakdown fats and proteins as well as promoting the health of the nervous system, skin, hair, eyes and importantly, the liver.

Vitamin B5 has a number of roles in the body some more critical than others. One job that is vitally important is assisting in the manufacture of red blood cells as well as sex and stress related hormones. Without B5 our digestive tract would become unhealthy and we would be unable to use other vitamins as effectively. It is sometimes referred to as the 'anti-stress' vitamin because it is believed to enhance the activity of the immune system and help the body overcome stressful conditions.

Currently research is looking into the benefits of B5 and treatment for elevated cholesterol but there are other areas where the vitamin may be beneficial.

Some studies are indicating that B5 may speed up wound healing especially following surgery and as part of a B-complex supplement it may help recovery from major burns. Arthritis has also come under the microscope as blood tests taken from arthritis sufferers' show that they were suffering from a deficiency of pantothenic acid, but more study will be needed to confirm this.

There are rumours that taking B5 can help with wrinkles and stop your hair greying but this is not proven.

What Are the Symptoms of a Deficiency?
If you are following a healthy eating plan with lots of fresh fruit, vegetables and whole grains you will be unlikely to be suffering from B5 deficiency.

If you were you might suffer from tiredness, headaches, nausea, tingling in the hands, depression, abdominal pains, insomnia, burning feet, muscle weakness and cramps. In extreme cases personality changes can take place as well as heart problems.

What Are the Dietary Sources of B5?
As we have pointed out, there are a large variety of sources for the vitamin including fresh meats, vegetables and whole grains. The best sources are Brewer's yeast, corn, cauliflower, broccoli,

tomatoes, avocado, lentils, egg yolks, organic beef, turkey, duck, chicken, milk, peanuts, soybeans, sunflower seeds, lobster, salmon and strawberries.

Most of the superfoods have really good amounts of the B vitamins and if they are included in your daily eating plan you should be getting more than adequate amounts.

If you are suffering from arthritis or depression seek the advice of a medical expert who can advise you on the dosage of any supplements including B5. If you take a multi-vitamin and mineral as I do, you will find that all the B vitamins are present and it is also sold separately under the names pantothenic acid and calcium pantothenate. In my experience it is easier to take in soft gel form as I find the tablets give me indigestion.

Vitamin B6: Pyridoxine

B6 is a water-soluble vitamin that exists in three major chemical forms: Pyridoxine, pyridoxal and pyridoxamine.

Being water soluble it is necessary to replace this vitamin every day from your diet and B6 plays such a crucial role in so many functions of the body that a deficiency can have a huge impact on your health.

It is required for over 100 enzymes that metabolise the protein that you eat. Along with the mineral Iron, it is essential for healthy blood and the nervous and immune systems require vitamin B6 to function efficiently. It is also necessary for our overall feeling of wellbeing as it converts the amino acid tryptophan, which is essential for the production of neurotransmitters such as serotonin in the brain.

Haemoglobin carries oxygen around the body in our blood and without B6 you would not be able to manufacture it in the first place. Additionally, once the haemoglobin is produced, the vitamin helps increase the amount of oxygen it can carry. A deficiency is therefore one of the leading causes of anaemia.

Without a healthy immune system we are at the mercy of any bacteria or virus that takes a fancy to us. A complicated biochemical interaction is required to ensure we can fight off infections and the food that we eat plays a vital role in producing the white blood cells that form the defence system. B6 ensures that the food that eat is metabolised efficiently thus producing enough of these cells. Additionally B6 helps keep your lymph system healthy by maintaining the thymus, spleen and lymph nodes. The lymph system runs parallel to your circulatory system and is the battleground for the white blood cells and the viruses.

Blood sugar levels can fluctuate depending on the types of food that we eat particularly carbohydrates. If you are not eating sufficient calories your body uses B6 to convert stored carbohydrate or other nutrients to glucose to maintain normal blood sugar levels. This is one of the reasons that people on crash diets can suffer dizziness and fatigue. Without sufficient intake of food they are not replenishing their B6 on a regular basis. Because they are taking in too little calories for their body to function and they do not have B6 to convert any stored energy, they become weakened.

The balance of chemicals in our brain affects our feeling of wellbeing. Neurotransmitters like serotonin, melatonin and dopamine are required for normal cell communication. In research lower levels of serotonin have been found in people suffering from varying degrees of depression and also migraine headaches. The research is not conclusive but as B6 is needed for the manufacture of these neurotransmitters it makes sense to ensure that there are adequate amounts being taken in through diet.

What Are the Other Signs of B6 Deficiency?

With a balanced diet, which includes whole grains and fruit and vegetables, it is unusual to find a B6 deficiency in a healthy adult. The elderly are more at risk due to reduced intakes of food resulting from lack of appetite and a general wearing down of internal systems and functions such as food metabolism. People who are perpetual dieters and in particular those who follow restricted food type diets are at risk as well, although unfortunately it is usually only when the deficiency has become critical that the symptoms might appear.

One of the early signs will be changes to the skin, with inflammations such as dermatitis. Another affected area is the mouth and Glossitis is a condition where the tongue becomes swollen and sore. Because of the role of B6 in our chemical balance within the brain, depression is not unusual. Alcoholics tend to eat poorly – which will restrict both their intake of B6 and its availability – but alcohol also causes the destruction and loss of any B6 that is consumed.

Taking too much vitamin B6 in supplementation form can

lead to some nerve damage particularly in the arms and legs. This might result in tingling sensations or numbness. Usually the symptoms disappear when the supplementation is stopped. Do talk to your doctor before stopping the supplement if you are taking it on his advice.

Best Food Sources for Vitamin B6

As always I prefer to include nutrients within our normal diet and as you will see from the healthy eating plan that there are many foods that you can include daily that will ensure that you have sufficient B6 for normal function. These foods include some of our superfoods like brown rice, walnuts, bananas, avocados, salmon as well as eggs, wheat germ, whole grains, poultry and meats such as lamb.

Vitamin B9: Folic Acid (Folate)

It is considered that this Vitamin is the most deficient in the World's population, which is a pretty frightening fact. Folic acid is fundamentally involved in the health of every single cell in our body and without it cells do not reproduce normally.

From the moment of conception Folic Acid ensures that the rapid reproduction of cells goes ahead without any defects. It is needed for the metabolism of RNA (ribonucleic acids) and DNA (deoxyribonucleic acids) in the cells' synthesis of protein. This is particularly important in the first twelve weeks of a foetus's existence and supplementation during this period is usually recommended. If a mother is suffering from a deficiency of the vitamin there is a very strong chance that the baby will be of a low birth weight and possibly have abnormalities such as heart problems or cleft palates.

Folic acid is also required for healthy blood formation and therefore reduces the risk of anaemia. It also helps boost the immune system particularly new babies.

It is essential for transporting co-enzymes needed for amino acid metabolism in the body and is necessary for a functioning nervous system.

Heart Disease

Heart disease is being linked to elevated levels of homocysteine an amino acid by-product in the blood. The B vitamins in general, but Vitamins B6, 12 and Folic Acid, have been shown to lower levels of this damaging substance and therefore reduce the risk of heart conditions developing.

It is involved in the health of the blood vessels and including high levels of folic acid rich foods can help reduce the risk of atherosclerosis, varicose veins and skin conditions such as psoriasis and eczema often the result of damaged capillaries under the skin.

Other Diseases That Folic Acid Is Linked To

A deficiency in Folic acid has been linked to a very varied number of diseases and conditions which makes the fact that it globally we are lacking in this vitamin all the more worrying. Some of these include breast, cervical, colon and lung cancer. Depression, schizophrenia and Alzheimer's disease – Digestive and bowel problems such as IBS, Celiac disease, ulcerative colitis and Crohn's disease – Skin conditions including psoriasis, eczema, dermatitis and skin ulcers.

Who Is Most Likely to Be Deficient in Folic Acid?

Unfortunately that could be anyone who does not include plenty of fresh dark green vegetables in their diet or whole grains, eggs and citrus fruits. In the Western world we are eating an increasingly whiter and more refined diet and combine this with excess sugars and processed foods and you have the potential for global deficiency.

Alcoholics are at risk as their bodies find it very difficult to process and absorb nutrients. The elderly have decreasing appetites and a less efficient digestive system as do people that rely heavily on antacids and frequent doses of over the counter medication.

There is some evidence to suggest that women who are taking either the contraceptive pill or HRT may also suffer from deficiencies and as pregnant women also are involved it would make sense that there might be a hormonal link to a lack of the vitamin.

What Are the Symptoms of a Folic Acid Deficiency?

The most common symptoms that could be present would be general fatigue, breathlessness, irritability, insomnia and forgetfulness.

What Are the Best Food Sources of Folic Acid?

All whole grains including brown rice and porridge oats, nuts, beans, dark green vegetables such as spinach and broccoli, offal as in liver and kidney and eggs.

Vitamin B12: Cynocolbalamin

B12 is an essential water-soluble vitamin but unlike other water soluble vitamins that are normally excreted in urine very quickly, B12 accumulates and gets stored in the liver (around 80%), kidney and body tissues. B12 is vital for the efficient working of every cell in the body especially those with a rapid turnover as it prevents cell degeneration. It functions as a methyl donor and works with folic acid in the manufacture of DNA and red blood cells and also is necessary to maintain the health of the insulating sheath (myelin sheath) that surrounds all nerve cells. It is involved in the production of melatonin, the hormone responsible for resetting our biological clock's rhythm when we change to new time zones, and also helps us sleep.

The most common disease associated with B12 deficiency is pernicious anaemia, which is characterised by large, immature red blood cells. But other diseases and medical conditions associated with a lack of this vitamin are allergies, Alzheimer's disease, asthma, cancer depression, AIDS, low blood pressure, multiple sclerosis, tinnitus and low sperm counts.

How Do We Become Deficient in B12?

We actually do not need a huge amount of the vitamin per day, around 2 micrograms or 2millionth of a gram. The problem is that it is not particularly well absorbed by the body so larger amounts are needed in the diet to supply the amount we need. Absorption of B12 requires the secretion from the cells lining the stomach of a glycoprotein, known as the intrinsic factor. The B12-intrinsic factor is then absorbed into the ileum (part of the small intestine) with calcium.

The problem we have today is that many people have turned away from the richest sources of B12 because they believe either that they are harmful, fattening or will raise levels of cholesterol. Liver, kidneys and eggs have not enjoyed wonderful press over the last few years and many people have also reduced the amount of cheese they eat believing that it is fattening.

Plant sources of B12 are virtually non-existent and many long term and dedicated vegetarians have been found to be deficient. Over use of antacids, inflammation of the stomach lining (Helicobacter pylori infection) and pancreatic problems can also lead to deficiency as the secretion of the intrinsic factor is compromised. There is some evidence that women with breast cancer have lower levels of B12 and there are indications that women after menopause with very low levels were more likely to develop the disease. It is not clear if the deficiency is caused by the cancer in the body or the other way around.

Some drugs have inhibited the uptake of B12 such as those prescribed for diabetes and ulcers and there is a great deal of research into these interactions.

As we age our ability to process our foods becomes less effective with enzyme production reduced such as the secretion of the intrinsic factor necessary for B12 absorption. Added to the fact that many elderly people suffer from a lack of appetite and you have a higher risk of malnutrition.

An interesting piece of research proposes that it is possible that Vitamin E may protect the process of absorption of B12 by preventing oxidative damage to cell membranes. If so a deficiency in this vitamin may well affect our B12 levels.

What Food Sources Are There for B12?

B12 is present in meats apart from offal, eggs and dairy products. It is better to drink a cold glass of milk than to eat yoghurt as the fermentation process destroys most of the B12 as does boiling milk. There are very few sources if any of B12 in plants although some people do believe that eating fermented Soya products, sea weeds and algae will provide the vitamin. However analysis of these products shows that whilst some of them do contain B12 it is in the form of B12 analogues which are unable to be absorbed by the human body.

Remember that eating foods containing Vitamin E may help the absorption process and the best sources for this are in nuts such as walnuts, sunflower seeds, whole grains, eggs, spinach, apples, bananas, broccoli, brown rice, carrots, onions and oily fish.

Most cereals and breads today are fortified with B12 as are yeast extracts (marmite) and vegetarian products.

Vitamin C: Ascorbate, Ascorbic Acid

We often take our vitamins for granted. The best way to take in Vitamin C is through the food that we eat, such as oranges. However, how many times when we are eating our oranges do we think about the over 300 biological processes in the body that Vitamin C is involved in.

Vitamin C or Ascorbic Acid is water-soluble and cannot be stored in the body. It therefore needs to be taken in through our food on a daily basis. It is in fact the body's most powerful water-soluble antioxidant and plays a vital role in protecting the body against oxidative damage from free radicals. It works by neutralising potentially harmful reactions in the water- based parts of our body such as the blood and within the fluids surrounding every cell. It helps prevent harmful cholesterol (LDL) from free radical damage, which can lead to plaque forming on the inside of arteries, blocking them. The antioxidant action protects the health or the heart, the brain and many other bodily tissues.

When we want to boost our immune system Vitamin C is an effective agent to use. It works by increasing the production of our white blood cells that make up our defence system, in particular B and T cells. It also increases levels of interferon and antibody responses improving antibacterial and antiviral effects. The overall effect is improved resistance to infection and it may also reduce the duration of the symptoms of colds for example. It may do this by reducing the blood levels of histamine, which has triggered the tissue inflammation and caused a runny nose. It has not been proven but certainly taking in vitamin C in the form of fruit and vegetable juices is not going to be harmful. Another affect may be protective as it prevents oxidative damage to the cells and tissues that occur when cells are fighting off infection.

This vitamin plays a role along with the B vitamins we have already covered in the conversion of tryptophan to serotonin, a neurotransmitter in the brain that helps determine our emotional well being.

Collagen is the protein that forms the basis of our connective tissue that is the most abundant tissue in the body. It glues cells together, supports and protects our organs, blood vessels, joints and muscles and also forms a major part of our skin, tendons, ligaments, corneas of the eye, cartilage, teeth and bone. Collagen also promotes healing of wounds, fractures and bruises. It is the degeneration of our collagen that leads to external signs of ageing such as wrinkles and sagging skin. There is a similar affect internally that can lead to degenerative diseases such as arthritis. Vitamin C is vital for the manufacture of collagen and is why taking in healthy amounts in your diet can combat the signs of ageing.

Our hormones require Vitamin C for the synthesis of hormones by the adrenal glands. These glands are situated above each kidney and are responsible for excreting the steroid hormones. The most important of these are aldosterone and cortisol. Cortisol regulates carbohydrate, protein and fat metabolism. Aldosterone regulates water and salt balance in the body and the other steroid hormones, of which there are 30; help counteract allergies, inflammation and other metabolic processes that are absolutely essential to life.

The cardiovascular system relies on Vitamin C that plays a role in cholesterol production in the liver and in the conversion of cholesterol into bile acids for excretion from the body. The vitamin also promotes normal total blood cholesterol and LDL (lousy cholesterol levels) and raises the levels of the more beneficial HDL (Healthy cholesterol) It supports healthy circulation and blood pressure, which in turn supports the heart.

The other areas that Vitamin C has shown it might be helpful to the body is in the lungs reducing breathing difficulties and improving lung and white blood cell function. It is recommended that smokers take Vitamin C not just in their diet but also as supplementation. Exposure to cigarette smoke may severely deplete the presence of Vitamin C in the lungs leading to cell damage.

Many studies are showing that Vitamin C can protect the health of the eye by possibly reducing ultra violet damage. The vitamin is very concentrated in the lenses of the normal eye which can contain up to 60 times more vitamin C than our blood. Damaged lenses appear to have a much lower amount of vitamin C which indicates that there is not sufficient to protect the lens from the effects of free radicals or support the enzymes in the lens that normally removed damaged cells.

Vitamin C works as part of a team helping in various metabolic processes such as the absorption of iron, converting folic acid to an active state, protecting against the effects of toxic effects of cadmium, copper, cobalt and mercury (brain health).

What Are the Signs of Deficiency of Vitamin C?

A total deficiency is extremely rare in the western World. A total lack of the vitamin leads to scurvy, which was responsible for thousands of deaths at sea from the Middle Ages well into the 19th century. Some voyages to the pacific resulted in a loss of as much as 75% of the crew. The symptoms were due to the degeneration of collagen that lead to broken blood vessels, bleeding gums, loose teeth, joint pains and dry scaly skin. Other symptoms were weakness, fluid retention, depression and anaemia. You can link these symptoms back up to the benefits of vitamin C and understand how many parts and processes of the body this vitamin is involved in.

In a milder form a deficiency has also been linked to increased infections, male infertility, rheumatoid arthritis and gastrointestinal disorders.

The best food source of vitamin C is all fresh, raw fruit and vegetables. Avoid buying prepared peeled and cut vegetables and fruit, as they will have lost the majority of their vitamin C. If you prepare juices at home, always drink within a few hours preferably immediately. Do not boil fruit and vegetables, it is better to eat raw whenever possible preserving all their nutrient content, but at the very least only steam lightly.

Researchers believe that taking in adequate amounts of Vitamin C is the best private health insurance that you can take out.

The best food sources is of course fresh fruit and vegetables but the highest concentrations are in Blackcurrants, broccoli, Brussel sprouts, cabbage, cauliflower, cherries, grapefruits, guavas, kiwi fruit, lemons, parsley, peppers, rosehips, potatoes, tomatoes and watercress.

Vitamin D: Cholecalciferol

If ever there was a reason to get out and lie in the sun for half the morning, getting your daily recommended dose of Vitamin D is it. In fact 3 hours in sunlight in moderate climates without using any sun block is sufficient to boost your levels of what is known as the sunshine vitamin. However, you do need less depending on latitude, time of day and air pollution.

It is not advisable to lie out in the heat of summer in Spain for example for 3 hours without protection but you will still receive beneficial amounts through sun block of under factor 8. Most of what we require on a daily basis is produced in the skin by the action of sunlight and many of us who suffer from depression through the dark winter months are actually missing around 75% of our required daily dose of 10ug.

There are a number of diseases that result from a deficiency of Vitamin D and over the years since it was identified in cod liver oil there has been increasing research into its role in the body.

In Victorian times children with rickets or bow legs were a common sight. You rarely see this in developed countries today although in Southern Asia there is still a problem. In adults the condition is called osteomalacia (soft bones) and it is estimated that millions of people who suffer from unexplained bone and muscle pain actually have this condition.

How Is Vitamin D Involved in Our Bones?

Our bones are living tissue that grows and regenerates throughout our lifetime. It is not static and old bone is removed and replaced with new bone continuously, a process that requires the essential elements of bone to be available from our diet and from chemical reactions in the body.

There are four main components in bone that are needed to ensure it is strong and able to repair itself on a daily basis.

- Minerals – calcium, magnesium and phosphorus.
- Matrix – collagen fibres (gristle)
- Osteoclasts – bone removing cells
- Osteoblasts – bone producing cells.

If you ever made paper Mâché sculptures at school you will have used a chicken wire framework first of all to establish the shape that you wanted. Over this you would have laid your strips of wet paper and allowed them to harden. The bone making process is very similar.

A network of collagen fibres form the base and they are then overlaid with minerals. The strength of the finished bone is dependent on the amount of mineralisation that takes place. Osteoclasts will remove old bone when needed and this results in a need to produce new collagen matrix to attract new minerals for the repair process.

Vitamin D is essential to ensure that sufficient calcium and phosphorus is attracted to the new matrix and that strong new bone is produced. Unfortunately if you are deficient in this vitamin more bone is discarded than replaced leading to soft and malformed bones.

Rickets for example is the result of soft and insufficient bone material in the legs allowing them to bend and stunting their growth. In adults the disease is called osteomalacia and because the symptoms are usually related to unspecific muscle and bone pain it can remain undiagnosed for years. This leads to chronic pain and the truth is that therapeutic doses of vitamin D may be the only treatment necessary.

Other Medical Problems Associated With Vitamin D Deficiency?

Arthritis is an autoimmune disease, which means that your own immune system is out of control and attacking your own tissues such as the joints. It has been known for some time that Vitamin D is necessary as part of the bone structure but it appears that it also works independently within the skeleton. It works its way into the lubricating synovial fluid inside joints and prevents the T-cells from the immune system attacking the tissues and causing inflammation. Research with Multiple Sclerosis another autoimmune disease is also showing this defensive action by vitamin D.

Cancer is the result of mutated cell growth into tumours and it is possible that vitamin D may regulate cell growth abnormalities, it is not clear if all cancers would respond to the vitamin but it will be interesting research to follow.

Vitamin D deficiency in our modern diet and the overuse of sun blocks over factor 8 is resulting in more and more incidences of Type 1 diabetes in children.

Hormonal fluctuations and problems such as PMS respond very well to calcium, magnesium and Vitamin D and I have worked with infertility related issues with clients who have also responded well to taking these three nutrients together. Calcium needs the vitamin to be absorbed so any process that involves the mineral will be more effective in combination including the management of blood sugar levels.

Phosphorus is not commonly deficient but as it requires Vitamin D to be absorbed in the first place it can become so. Phosphorus is involved in a number of functions other than bone production including the production of energy, enzyme processes, activation of B complex vitamins and keeping the blood alkaline. If we are therefore deficient in Vitamin D we are affecting all these essential functions within the body.

Many people suffer from Seasonal Affective Disorder (SAD) and I have to say that if I go more than a few days without some sunshine I can begin to feel less energetic and more irritable. Vitamin D treatment has been highly successful in this area although the use of light boxes, as a form of therapy has not been as effective. Obviously you either need to supplement or get out into some real daylight.

There are links to a number of other medical issues including obesity and it is going to be interesting to see what research is going to discover about this particular vitamin in years to come.

What Are the Best Sources for Vitamin D?

A walk in the fresh air is great for you and for those of us in Spain or other Mediterranean countries we have the added bonus of sunshine. Try to walk in the cooler mornings without any sun block or at least keep to under factor 8 at least 5 times per week. You can walk again in the evening for an hour before sunset. This way you will lose weight, tone up, get lightly tanned and get your daily Vitamin D.

My theory is that we evolved into obtaining this essential nutrient from the sun because there were not sufficient food sources for it. We need at least 10ug per day and we need to include oily fish and eggs regularly to obtain sufficient. Eggs contain approximately 1ug with a 100 gm serving of herring or tinned salmon providing the maximum at 16.5 μg. Vegetarians and Vegans need to eat fortified cereals to obtain enough vitamin D and usually they are the most at risk of deficiency diseases. Taking cod liver oil capsules is an excellent way to get your Vitamin D, which is probably why it is also an effective preventative and support for rheumatoid arthritis.

As we get older our skin thins and we are less able to manufacture Vitamin D naturally, which is when supplementation is a good idea. It is a good idea to take not only cod liver oil but also an additional supplement of calcium, magnesium and Vitamin D.

Vitamin E: Tocopherol

Vitamin E is a powerful antioxidant that helps protect the body from free radical damage to nerve and cell membranes. It works within the body to protect the more harmful cholesterol (LDL) from free radical damage and therefore helps prevent the build up of plaque leading to atherosclerosis. As you will have read from the chapter on heart disease, atherosclerosis is the leading cause of heart problems and including vitamin E rich foods in your diet is very important as part of the battle to keep your arteries healthy.

There is a great deal of research currently being conducted into the benefits of vitamin E and these include studies into cancer prevention, diabetes, Alzheimer's disease, fibrocystic breast disease and cataracts.

In the circulatory system is appears to prevent clots from forming which is the leading cause of strokes and it also improves the function of the lungs. You will find it as an active ingredient in many skin preparations from cosmetics to topical creams for skin conditions. It is very effective when teamed up with the healing properties of zinc.

Our immune system function is our first line of defence against bacteria and viral infections and this vitamin is very important in maintaining the integrity of the white blood cells.

I have designed eating programmes for women for many years and have always included vitamin E rich foods as it can help with PMS, menopausal symptoms and keep the reproductive system healthy especially during pregnancy.

Athletes will find that eating vitamin E rich foods will also help repair muscles and protect them from free radical damage and can also reduce the level of inflammation and soreness associated with very active lifestyles.

So to sum up, Vitamin E is a very valuable ally in the fight against not only disease but also ageing and it is present in a great many of everyday foods making it easy to include in our diet.

VITAMIN E

- Improves immunity and helps you look younger internally and externally.
- Protects polyunsaturated fats from free radical damage
- Improves body's oxygen supply for more energy/endurance
- Helps white blood cells to resist infection
- Protects against cancer
- Protects against thrombosis, heart attacks and strokes
- Increases 'good' cholesterol and protects 'bad' cholesterol from free radical damage

- Speeds up healing of burns
- Helps to reduce risk of miscarriage
- Works with selenium as a combined antioxidant

What Are the Deficiency Symptoms of Vitamin E?

In children you might notice increase irritability, water retention and unusual tiredness. In adults apart from lack of energy there might also be poor concentration, loss of sex drive and some muscle weakness.

Are There Any Side Effects From Taking Supplemental Vitamin E?

It is always a good idea to obtain as many of your nutrients from your food as possible, but vitamin E is often taken as we get older for many of the reasons we have already discussed.

There is some toxic reaction to vitamin E if it is taken in excess in the form of muscle weakness but doctors have prescribed 5,000 IU for patients with no ill effects. The normal supplemental dose is between 100 IU and 800 IU per day and I would advise that you should not exceed 400 IU per day without the supervision of your doctor.

Ideally you will be obtaining sufficient vitamin E from the foods included in your diet.

Vitamin E is fat soluble and found in nuts such as almonds and walnuts, sunflower seeds and their oil, whole grains like maize, egg yolks and leafy green vegetables like spinach. Also found in apples, bananas, broccoli, brown rice, carrots, lamb's liver, onions, Sunflower oil, oily fish and shellfish.

Vitamin K: Phylloquinone

There are two forms of the vitamin that the body can utilise. One is K1 (phylloquinone), which is from plant sources and the other is K2 (menaquinone) which is produced by bacteria in our own intestines. This is where many of us get into trouble because we are not eating sufficient raw and unprocessed foods for health and additionally many of us suffer from bacterial imbalances in the gut so do not produce sufficient from that source either.

The vitamin is fat-soluble and is stored in the liver. Studies indicate that approximately 50% of the stores come from our diet and the balance from bacteria in the intestines. We need healthy bile production for efficient absorption of Vitamin K and our lymphatic system circulates it throughout the body.

Apart from helping reduce excessive bleeding during menstruation it is also used therapeutically for the prevention of internal bleeding and haemorrhages including emergency treatment for overdoses of blood thinners such as Warfarin.

Blood clotting is a critical function in the body that solidifies blood to prevent us from bleeding to death from external or internal injuries. Vitamin K is essential for the production of a protein called prothrombin and other factors involved in the blood-clotting function and are therefore necessary to prevent haemorrhages. Also interestingly Vitamin K also activates other enzymes that decrease the clotting ability so it assumes the role of regulator within the bloodstream. An example of this might be if a clot forms within a blood vessel that could block the flow and needs to be dispersed.

The vitamin has also been the subject of a great deal of research in recent years as scientists discovered that it played a significant role in liver function, energy production in the nervous system and in preventing bone loss as we age by assisting the absorption of calcium.

Vitamin K is needed to activate osteocalcin, the protein that anchors calcium into the bone, building and repairing the structure. A deficiency in the vitamin can therefore lead to brittle bones and osteoporosis.

As the vitamin works within the body it changes from function to function according to the various interactions with enzymes and at one stage it acts as an antioxidant preventing oxidative damage to cells. There may also be a role for the vitamin in cancer prevention as it is believed it may stimulate rogue cells to self destruct.

Why Are You Likely to Be Deficient?

As I mentioned above if you do not include sufficient Vitamin K rich foods in your diet then you will be missing out on 50% of your requirements immediately. If you have prolonged use of anti-biotics you will have compromised the bacterial balance in your intestines and reduced the production of the vitamin from this source too.

Anyone suffering from gall bladder or liver disease may well suffer a deficiency as do people with malabsorption problems such as celiac disease. Newborn babies are often given vitamin K particularly if they are going to be breast fed and the mother is deficient and anyone taking anti-coagulant drugs such as Warfarin or Dicoumarol will find that these block the effect of the vitamin.

Some people might be susceptible to deficiency if they are taking high amounts of Vitamin A and E as these can block the absorption of Vitamin K. A slightly acidic environment is necessary for the efficient production of this vitamin so people who use antacids on a very regular basis neutralise their stomach acid resulting in neutralised chyme (stomach contents) passing into the duodenum.

What Are the Symptoms of Vitamin K Deficiency?

Men and women who find that their blood fails to clot after an injury are also likely candidates as well as people who suffer from frequent and heavy nosebleeds.

Other symptoms include eye haemorrhages, anaemia, bleeding gums, easy bruising, frequent fractures and other bone problems.

What Are the Best Food Sources for Vitamin K?

It is very easy to obtain sufficient Vitamin K through diet and you will good sources in dark green leafy vegetables such as asparagus, avocado, broccoli, Brussel sprouts, green beans as well as carrots and eggs.

Although the vitamin is fairly resilient it is better to eat plant sources either raw or lightly steamed to obtain the maximum benefits. Freezing reduces the amount of the vitamin so you need to eat a little extra of frozen vegetables than fresh.

Coenzyme Q10: Ubiquinone

As with many supplements there are advocates and sceptics and Coenzyme Q10 is no exception. There are many people however, who take Q10 on a daily basis that feel that this "vitamin" is a super nutrient.

I personally take Q10 and can only say that I feel a difference when I do not take it on a regular basis which is the way that I determine if a supplement is actually doing me any good. As with any supplement, results tend not to happen overnight and my body seems to take about a month to register any marked improvements.

Many people believe that Q10 can slow the progress of Parkinson's disease, stabilise blood sugar levels in diabetics, improve circulation and stamina as well as prevent degenerative diseases of the eye. There is some question as to whether taking the nutrient in supplemental form is actually as effective as claimed but there is evidence, which shows that taking Q10 can support the heart.

What Is Coenzyme Q10?

The body actually naturally produces this compound and it is found in every human cell as well as in most foods in small amounts.

It is a member of a family of compounds called quinones and because it primarily works with enzymes in the body it is called coenzyme Q10. It is particularly abundant in cells of the body that require a great deal of energy such as the heart muscle and it also works as an extremely powerful antioxidant preventing free radical damage.

What Are The Researched Health Benefits of Q10?

CONGESTIVE HEART FAILURE

In certain countries such as Canada, Sweden and Japan, a large proportion of the population with heart problems takes Q10. There is evidence to support supplementation in cases of congestive heart failure and blocked arteries and in a recent study there was definitely a reduction in accompanying symptoms. Over 80% of the 2,500 members of the trial experienced a reduction in swollen ankles, breathing difficulties and sleep problems. It did not cure the problem but certainly improved the quality of life for the sufferers.

There have been other studies that have not shown quite such a clear cut benefit from taking Q10 but I feel that so many of these studies are not conclusive anyway as so many other factors are simply not taken into consideration.

ANGINA AND ARRHYTHMIAS

There is evidence to suggest that taking Q10 might reduce the frequency of painful angina attacks and also relieve the stress on the heart helping to stabilise heart rhythms.

CANCER

Several studies have indicated that taking Q10 may help prevent and treat cancers of the prostate and breast. There is no clear explanation as yet but it is believed that the antioxidant effect of

Q10 may boost the body's own immune system thereby limiting the spread of the cancerous cells.

HIGH BLOOD PRESSURE.
It is thought that over 35% of patients with very high blood pressure are deficient in Q10 and that by taking a supplement on a daily basis they may help lower not only the blood pressure but also help protect themselves from the effects of the disease.

DEGENERATIVE BRAIN DISEASE
Some interesting studies are being conducted on Alzheimer's disease and the possible benefit of anyone over the age of 50 taking Q10 as a supplement. It is thought to slow down the progression of the disease, possibly due to its antioxidant effect on the brain cells. There is certainly a reduction in the body's own production of Q10 once we get into middle age and apart from increasing energy levels as we age it may well also help us hang onto our short term memories.

Q10 AND CHOLESTEROL LOWERING DRUGS
Prescribed medication such as Statins for high cholesterol levels not only restrict the production of cholesterol by the liver but also block the production of Coenzyme Q10. As Q10 is so important to the body in a great many ways it would seem sensible to supplement with the nutrient when taking these drugs.

What Are the Other Reasons for Taking Q10?
Around the world millions of people are taking Q10 for a host of reasons apart from the ones that I have already mentioned. These include anti-ageing, Chronic Fatigue, Fibrosis, Fibromyalgia, Male Infertility, Multiple sclerosis, Skin health and Weight loss.

It can be expensive so it is best to shop around and as always if you are taking any prescribed medication for blood pressure or heart disease do talk to your doctor first.

Minerals

Calcium

This is the most abundant and essential mineral in the body. There are about two or three pounds of calcium, which is mainly found in the teeth and the bones. Apart from the more obvious role in the formation of teeth and bones it is also essential for the efficiency in many of our other body systems such as blood clotting, transmission of signals in our nerve cells and our muscle contractions.

Like all nutrients there is a great deal of research being conducted into the various ways that calcium works within our bodies and our precise requirement for it. There is some indication that a higher intake of calcium can protect against cardiovascular disease, mainly in women.

If you are at risk from kidney stones you need to be careful about taking in calcium supplements and this also applies when taking in additional dietary calcium in the form of dairy products if you are suffering from prostate cancer. One of the reasons for this is that excess calcium depletes the body of Vitamin D, which is known to protect against prostate cancer.

The best dietary sources of calcium are through eating moderate amounts of dairy products, sardines and canned salmon with the bones, green leafy vegetables such as spinach and soy products such as tofu.

Chromium

Chromium is an essential trace mineral that helps the body maintain normal blood sugar levels. A deficiency of the mineral can lead to Diabetes and this is where the primary research into this mineral has been directed.

Chromium first and foremost is a component of the 'glucose tolerance factor' which is required for maintaining a normal blood glucose balance. Chromium works with insulin to ease the absorption of blood glucose into the cells and it may also play a part in other activities that involve insulin such as the metabolism of fats and proteins.

This last activity has opened a line of research in the effect of chromium on weight loss, building muscle and decreasing body fat and has led to a lot of chromium based products being put on the market in recent years. There is no definite proof that it works although some studies do claim that in a study that people on chromium lost more body fat over three months than those who did not take it.

It is more important to look at the role of chromium as we age as there is increasing numbers of patients who are diagnosed with late onset Diabetes. This is nearly always related to dietary deficiency and the concern is that with our current trend towards eating processed foods and excess weight are responsible as we are automatically taking in less chromium in raw and unprocessed foods.

Chromium is very easy to lose from the body in urine, sweat and if we engage in excessive physical activity without the appropriate diet. However, chromium is very easy to include in any healthy diet and should not be needed in supplement form. If you are a diabetic then you must make sure that you work with your medical advisor before taking any chromium supplement, as it will affect the dosage of any insulin you may be taking.

Other areas that chromium may have an influence on your health are with elevated blood pressure, high cholesterol and low HDL (High-density lipoproteins or Healthy cholesterol) in your blood.

What Are the Best Food Sources for Chromium

Best food sources for chromium are; whole grains, potatoes, oysters, liver, seafood, cheese, chicken, turkey, beef, lamb and pork. Dark leafy vegetables such as broccoli and romaine lettuce contain healthy amounts as do onions and tomatoes.

Copper

Copper is the third most abundant trace mineral in the body but as the best food sources are oysters and liver, most of us get too little of this vital nutrient.

Copper has numerous functions within the body and is a component in many of the chemical processes. We often associate the colour copper with blood and in fact it is involved in the formation of haemoglobin and red blood cells. Pigmentation of our hair and skin is dependent on the mineral and it works with Vitamin C to produce collagen for bone, connective tissues and the skin.

It is necessary for healthy heart function, helping to regulate the pumping action and it also helps control cholesterol and sugar levels as well as the amount of uric acid in our bloodstream.

As an adult we would contain between 100 and 150 mg, the majority in the skeleton and the muscles. Some is stored in the liver until mixed with bile and secreted into the intestines to be disposed of and there are sizeable amounts in the brain, kidneys and heart. Babies have ten times the copper than adults in their livers as there is barely any present in breast milk. This is a sure indicator of how necessary this particular mineral is to our general health.

Specific Roles of Copper in The Body
THE HEART
In order to pump blood around the body a steady and sustained rhythm is necessary from the heart muscle. Copper helps regulate not only irregular heart beats (arrhythmia) but helps reduce elevated cholesterol levels too, preventing a build up of plaque that leads to raised blood pressure levels and subsequent heart disease.

EYE, SKIN AND HAIR COLOUR
Our hair and skin colour depends on melanin and copper is a major component of this pigment. It influences the colour of our eyes, how dark our skin is and prevents our hair from losing its natural colour and turning grey. It is said that taking copper supplements can restore your hair colour from grey but I would suggest that you read the side effects before throwing away your Clairol.

RHEUMATOID ARTHRITIS
You will often see people wearing copper bracelets to alleviate rheumatism symptoms and this is a centuries old remedy as copper is absorbed through the skin. However, it is a bit hit and miss and taking copper supplements in a regulated dose is actually more effective. As rheumatoid arthritis sufferers also tend to be deficient in zinc you will often find the two supplements combined for better effectiveness.

Copper Deficiency Symptoms

It is not usual to be suffering from a deficiency of copper in the western World but some of the indications are anaemia, water retention, irritability, frequent fractures, loss of hair colour and texture and a loss of sense of taste.

People on highly processed diets will likely be lacking in copper as will anybody suffering from malabsorption problems or prolonged diarrhoea. There is a specific disease, which is called Menke's syndrome where lack of copper leads to connective tissue and bone damage and this is a genetic disease mainly effecting baby boys with females being the carriers.

Side Effects

If you are taking in more than 10 mg per day you could begin to suffer from stomach cramps, nausea, muscle pain and possible diarrhoea so do be aware when taking additional copper supplements.

What Are the Best Food Sources for Copper?

As I mentioned before, many people have moved away from eating animal offal, which is a shame as it is a very rich source for many essential nutrients. Liver is full of copper but if you cannot bring yourself to enjoy this with onions and bacon then include shell fish, olives, nuts, beans, wholegrain cereals, dried fruits, meat, fish and poultry regularly in your diet.

Iodine

Iodine's role in the body is specifically within the thyroid gland at the base of the neck and as a component of the thyroid hormones in the blood, triiodothyronine and thyroxine. The role of these hormones is to determine the level of metabolism in the body or if you like the speed at which our operating systems work.

Iodine in our diet is converted into iodide in the intestines and then carried into general circulation by serum proteins. As soon as it reaches the thyroid gland it is trapped and stored to manufacture the thyroid hormones, thyroxine and triiodothyronine. These hormones regulate cell activity and growth in nearly all of our tissues and are therefore particularly important during the development of a foetus.

They also regulate how fast we live which means that they regulate our metabolism, which converts food into energy and also the rate at which that energy is dispersed.

There are parts of the world that are known as "goitre belts" and this refers to the high incidence of neck goitres a physical symptom of an under active thyroid gland due to a deficiency in iodine. The cause is usually poorly mineralised soil creating deficient amounts in crops. In the UK there was an expression called "Derbyshire Neck" because so many people in that county suffered from the disease.

Iodine deficiency is actually a worldwide medical epidemic with certain countries such as Africa, India and China suffering the most. A combination of poor soil quality and over population that is reliant on local produce is a recipe for a number of iodine related diseases.

If a foetus does not receive sufficient iodine through its mother's diet it is at an increased risk of mental defects due to impaired physical growth and neurological development which can damage the brain. The damage can range from mild speech or movement problems to severe retardation and it is estimated that if affects almost a third of the 1.5 billion people in the world who are living in this nutritionally depleted environment. Even European countries are at risk if they are mountainous as water from glaciers or heavy rainfall areas wash the mineral from the soil. Switzerland has some communities that have a high incidence of iodine deficiency related conditions. Another problem is the reliance of localised communities on food grown in their area which means that how ever diversified their food range is all of it will be affected by the lack of iodine in the soil. Some people that rely heavily on one specific food source are also at risk as certain foods such as cabbage, Brussel sprouts, legumes and cassava contain a substance that blocks the absorption of any iodine that is present resulting in deficiencies.

That means that over 50 million people are affected by the lack of one mineral in their diet and puts Avian Flu and Mad Cow disease into perspective.

What Are the Deficiency Symptoms for Iodine?

If a person is suffering from too little iodine they are likely to suffer from weight gain, fatigue, muscle weakness, coarse skin and drowsiness. Unfortunately this reflects the symptoms of many nutritionally related diseases and this is why any healthy eating plan should contain such a wide variety of foods from as many different sources as possible.

What Are the Best Food Sources for Iodine?

The best food sources are found in seafood and sea vegetables such as kelp. An easy way to ensure adequate amounts is by using iodised salt, which is available in most supermarkets and health food shops. Eating fish such as cod, mackerel and haddock is great and you will find good sources in eggs, low fat live yoghurt, milk and strawberries.

Iron

Iron is vital to the health of the entire human body and is present in every cell. It is part of haemoglobin the oxygen-carrying component of the blood and normally the body would contain around 4 grams of iron. Iron is also a component of myoglobin, which distributes and helps muscle cells store oxygen. Without iron the Adenosine Triphosphate (ATP the fuel we run on) could not be produced and long term this is very serious.

Dietary iron is found in two forms, heme iron and non-heme iron. Heme iron, which is the most absorbable, is found only in animal flesh as it is taken from the haemoglobin and myoglobin in animal tissue. Non-heme iron is found in plant foods and dairy products.

Other duties that are performed by iron include the production of energy as a component of a number of enzymes and it is also involved in the production of the nonessential amino acid, L-Carnitine, important for the efficient metabolism of fat.

Who Might Be Deficient in Iron?

Our bodies are very efficient at processing iron from food and old red blood cells to fulfil its needs, but if there is insufficient in our diet in the first place, then over a period of time we will become iron deficient.

If you have a balanced diet of lean meat, fruit and vegetables this is unlikely to happen unless you have an underlying medical condition or you are leading an extremely active lifestyle.

Vegetarians will be consuming non-heme iron from plant sources and this is less absorbable and therefore they are likely to have a reduced store of the mineral. This in itself is not a problem if iron rich foods are included regularly in the diet, but women who are vegetarians should increase iron intake during and after periods, particularly if they are heavy. This could also apply to regular blood donors.

Others who might have reduced stores of iron are pregnant women, young children that are growing rapidly, high performance athletes, anyone with a gastrointestinal problem or a parasitic condition such as Candida.

Supplementation of iron does not work for everyone and in fact it is linked to certain problems such as constipation and it can be dangerous for people with conditions such as Hemochromatosis (excess storage of iron in the liver) or sickle cell anaemia.

Certain foods and supplements restrict the absorption of iron such as caffeine, antacids and calcium supplements. Drinking excessive amounts of carbonated soft drinks can also effect your iron absorption and it is a particular problem with teenagers especially girls who have begun their periods. Excessive alcohol will also affect absorption of iron resulting in deficiency symptoms. If you are taking iron supplements you should always take at least a couple hours before or after a cup of tea. Conversely Vitamin A rich foods help the body utilise the iron that is stored in the liver

What Are Some of the Signs of an Iron Deficiency?
The first likely symptom is extreme fatigue. Without sufficient iron, underdeveloped red blood cells, lacking correct levels of haemoglobin, will be unable to carry enough oxygen to all the cells in the body. There might be weakness, loss of stamina, breathlessness, infections, hair loss, dizziness and brittle nails. It is not unusual to find that people who suffer from depression are also iron deficient. Young children may suffer from learning disabilities and behavioural problems.

Anyone suffering from iron deficiency anaemia, leukaemia, stomach ulcers, tuberculosis, colitis and alcoholism will need to supplement with iron under the direction of their medical advisor.

What Are the Best Food Sources for Iron?
For the rest of us we need to include a range of seafood, including cockles, mussels and clams; liver; kidneys; prunes; spinach; meats; wheat-germ and cocoa in our diet. Drinking and eating high

Vitamin C content foods at the same time may help your body absorb iron more efficiently.

Magnesium

One of the minerals that most people focus on is calcium but it is in fact magnesium or the lack of this mineral in our diet that may be the contributory factor in many of the diseases that we suffer from, particularly as we get older.

It is believed that the availability of magnesium in drinking water and in our soil is now greatly decreased. Not only is the soil depleted but the plants that we eat are also becoming more and more magnesium deficient for two reasons. There is less magnesium in the soil that nourishes them and the use of potassium and phosphorus-laden fertilisers alter the ability of the plant to absorb the mineral. When we cook food we lose magnesium and if we restrict our calories during a diet or eat high carbohydrate and fat diets we increase the risks associated with deficiency.

It is staggering how many diseases are linked to a deficiency of this mineral including Alzheimer's, angina, asthma, autism, auto immune disorders, congestive heart failure, depression, diabetes, eating disorders such as bulimia and anorexia, heart disease, high blood pressure, kidney stones, Multiple sclerosis, muscle weakness, Parkinson's disease and osteoporosis.

Magnesium works with calcium in a number of ways. Calcium causes muscles to contract and magnesium to relax. It is needed to balance calcium in the body and a deficiency can result in bone calcium being leached from the bones.

Magnesium plays a role in a number of critical functions within the body. It is essential for the transmission of hormones such as the secretion and action of insulin, thyroid and oestrogen and in the neurotransmitters such as serotonin. It is needed for bone, protein and fatty acid formation, forming new cells, activating the B vitamins, clotting blood and helping form the ATP (Adenosine Triphosphate) fuel that we run on.

Magnesium is also essential to protect us against heavy metal poisoning and a deficiency has been linked to these metals being deposited in the brain leading to Alzheimer's and other brain disorders.

There are a number of risk factors that decrease our ability to absorb magnesium including excessive alcohol intake, using recreational drugs, excessive levels of calcium, too much caffeine in coffee, severe dieting, high intake of phosphorus laden foods such as fizzy drinks and processed foods. Too much salt in the diet, over exercising and physical and mental stress also contribute.

What Are the Best Food Sources for Magnesium?

The best food sources for magnesium are dairy products, fish, meat, seafood, apples, apricots, avocados, bananas, whole grain cereals such as brown rice, nuts, dark green vegetables such as spinach and also mineral water.

Manganese

Manganese is a macro mineral or trace element that is essential for the normal formation of bone and cartilage. It is also necessary for efficient metabolism of glucose and forms part of the antioxidant super oxide dismutase.

Unfortunately only about 5% of dietary manganese is absorbed which means that adequate amounts need to be taken in on a daily basis in our food.

It is involved in a number of production processes including energy production, healthy joints, immune system function, sex hormones and thyroxine one of the hormones produced by the thyroid gland. Without thyroxine our metabolism would be inefficient and there would be an affect on every aspect of our health.

There are certain diseases where tests have shown the patients have been deficient in manganese and these include diabetes, heart disease, atherosclerosis, rheumatoid arthritis and mental conditions such as schizophrenia.

What Is the Role of Manganese in Bone Health?

We tend to think of calcium and magnesium being the major bone minerals but in fact manganese and one of the main nutrients in Spinach, Vitamin K is also absolutely essential to ensure healthy bones.

Bone is not a solid substance, it is a living and changing tissue that not only provides the structural framework for our bodies but is also used to protect major organs such as the brain, spinal cord and the nursery for blood vessels.

We all made plaster or paper Mâché sculptures at school and would have begun with a framework and some form of mesh, usually made from chicken wire. In the body this mesh is called the osteoid and is made up of protein, collagen, elastin and Glucosamine polymers. New bone is being produced all the time, particularly if there are breaks or wear and tear so this mesh requires certain nutrients in our diet all the time including Vitamin C for collagen and B6, copper and zinc. The Glucosamine polymers also contain manganese and to effectively combine all these components you need Vitamin K.

Once the network is in place calcium and magnesium have a framework that they can attach themselves to and bone is formed.

What Other Roles Does Manganese Play in the Body?

The body's operating systems have a workforce made up of enzymes. Enzymes are protein based molecules that speed up all the chemical processes in the body or acts as a catalyst for a particular function. For example without enzymes, digestion of food would not happen and we would be starved of the nutrients we need to survive. Without enzymes we could not live.

Manganese plays a role in most major enzyme activities in the body by activating certain nutrients necessary to the process such as biotin (manufacture of glycogen and prostaglandins in the immune system), thiamin, Vitamin C (immune system) and Choline (essential neurotransmitter in the brain). It is also involved in the synthesis or fatty acids and cholesterol, is involved in the processing of protein and carbohydrates and is involved in the manufacture of some hormones. Therefore manganese helps maintain normal blood sugar levels, thyroid function, cholesterol levels, a healthy nervous system and acts as an antioxidant.

What Are the Symptoms of Deficiency for Manganese?

If someone is suffering from pre-diabetes and has elevated blood sugar levels they are likely to be deficient in manganese in their diet. In extreme cases they may suffer from nausea and vomiting, skin rashes, dizziness and hearing loss. It is internally however that the real damage may be occurring and that is in extensive bone loss that might only be identified in late middle age.

What Health Issues Are Linked to Manganese?

Considering manganese is not often referred to it is involved in the treatment or prevention of a number of conditions, including asthma. It also plays a role in diabetes, epilepsy, heart disease, osteoporosis, rheumatoid arthritis, PMS and brain disorders.

What Are the Best Food Sources for Manganese?

Thankfully there are plenty of delicious food sources for this mineral and they should all be included regularly in a healthy eating plan. Beans are an alternative source of protein but they also contain a healthy amount of manganese, as do spinach, brown rice, tomatoes and walnuts.

Other foods that need to be included in your diet are asparagus, pineapples, whole grains, porridge oats, dark green leafy vegetables, raspberries and strawberries. It is also in herbs and spices such as basil, cloves, cinnamon, thyme, black pepper and oregano.

Anyone, who has a healthy diet comprising plenty of fresh fruit and vegetables, whole grains and herbal teas, will be getting adequate amounts of manganese in their diets. If you are taking a good quality multi-vitamin and mineral you will find that it will also be included in the formula which will give you a back up in times of infection or stress.

Phosphorus

Phosphorus is a mineral that you will not find in your multi-vitamin and mineral supplement because it is considered that we obtain sufficient through our diet.

However there are some interesting facts about phosphorus that makes it worth taking a closer look at. Many women as they approach the menopause will begin to supplement with additional calcium to prevent bone loss and take up weight bearing exercise such as walking and yoga. However, very few women and men too realise that phosphorus is also very important for bone health and without it calcium is less effective.

Clinical studies have shown that calcium supplementation without enough phosphorus may actually lead to bone mass reduction. Although most calcium supplements are combined with Vitamin D to assist absorption, trials have shown that with the addition of phosphorus bone fractures in high-risk patients was reduced by 43% within 18 months.

One doctor said that they are like bricks and mortar and you can only build a healthy and strong bone structure with the two of them in the correct proportion.

What Is Phosphorus?

Phosphorus is an essential mineral usually combined with oxygen as a phosphate. Most phosphate in the body is found in our bones. But, phosphate containing molecules, (phospholipids) are also important components of cell membranes and lipoprotein particles such as HDL (healthy cholesterol) and LDL (lousy cholesterol). A small amount of phosphate plays a role in many of our biochemical reactions including the production of our essential fuel ATP (adenosine triphosphate) and the formation of red blood cells.

What Are the Signs of Deficiency for Phosphorus?

Deficiency is rare in a person with a normal diet. Alcoholics however are at risk as are people who are constantly taking antacids because of the aluminium content in some brands. Osteoporosis sufferers who are heavily supplementing with calcium are also at risk of deficiency and it is usually recommended that they take phosphorus at the same time.

The far bigger risk with phosphorus is the amount we are consuming in processed foods such as soft drinks. A diet high in phosphorus may decrease the absorption of other minerals such as iron, copper and zinc.

Phosphoric acid for example in soft drinks has been linked to kidney stones in some trials and certainly people with kidney disease should avoid taking in any food or drink that contains excessive amounts of the mineral.

What Are the Best Food Sources for Phosphorus?

Sufficient phosphorus is found in a diet that includes plenty of protein rich foods such as turkey and other poultry and meats. Vegetarians need to include plenty of whole grains in their diet to ensure that they obtain sufficient phosphorus.

Potassium

Potassium (K) is the most essential cation (positively charged electrolyte.) It reacts with sodium and chloride to maintain a perfect working environment in and around each cell.

It is necessary for normal kidney function and it also plays a part in heart and bone health with a particular role in smooth muscle contraction. The heart muscle must maintain a smooth and regular heartbeat and correct levels of potassium in the body will help regulate this. Some studies are indicating that low dietary potassium intake is linked to high blood pressure and that combined with calcium and magnesium rich foods can go a long way to preventing this condition from developing. A balance of potassium, calcium and magnesium is essential to maintain bone mass and a deficiency is linked to osteoporosis.

Who Might Be Deficient in Potassium?
With a normal healthy and balanced diet with plenty of fresh fruit and vegetables there should be no reason for a person to be deficient in potassium. The elderly are more at risk, as total body potassium levels deplete with age. Also anyone who is taking certain prescribed medication may find their potassium levels dropping, particularly if they are taking nonsteroidal anti-inflammatories (NSAIDs) or ACE inhibitors for high blood pressure. Taking over the counter medication such as antacids or laxatives can also cause a loss of too much potassium. Insulin is another drug that can cause a decrease in potassium and therefore diabetics must watch their diet carefully to ensure that they are receiving sufficient.

There are occasional problems that might deplete the mineral's stores such as a stomach upsets with diarrhoea and vomiting, excessive exercise resulting in heavy sweating, crash dieting and taking diuretics. Drinking lots of tea and coffee can also increase the amount of potassium excreted in the urine. It is important that you take in sufficient amounts of magnesium rich foods to balance the levels of potassium in the body.

What Happens If Potassium Is Out of Balance in the Body?
If you have too much potassium in your blood it is called hyperkalemia and too little is called hypokalemia.

Hyperkalemia might be caused by a number of factors including suffering severe burns, undergoing chemotherapy or severe muscle loss through illness. There are a number of conditions that inhibit the normal excretion of potassium in the urine and these include kidney failure and a problem with the adrenal glands. The adrenal gland makes a hormone called aldosterone that signals the body to excrete or conserve potassium based on the body's needs and in hyperkalemia there may be fewer hormones produced or excreted.

Symptoms of too much potassium in your blood might be tingling in fingers and toes, muscle weakness and numbness. It can lead to irregular heartbeats and further heart problems if not treated.

Hypokalemia is more common as this is often dietary related as we have mentioned above. It can also be a result of a problem in the adrenal glands but in this case it is when the hormone aldosterone is retained causing the kidneys to conserve the potassium instead of excreting it.

The symptoms of too little potassium would include muscle pain, irritability, weakness and possibly paralysis.

There are some studies that are linking deficiency of potassium to a number of medical conditions including increased risk of stroke. Certainly in patients who already have elevated blood pressure, including dietary potassium seems to reduce the risk of stroke but not apparently if it is given in supplementation form. Another condition, which can result in potassium deficiency, is Inflammatory Bowel disease such as colitis or Crohn's disease. In this case it is usual to supplement with the mineral but only under medical supervision. A diet high in potassium will help, as foods like banana are also very soothing for intestinal problems.

Other studies show that children who suffer from asthma and therefore have poor lung function may have diets that are too low in potassium and there may be an improvement by increasing the amounts of fresh fruit, vegetables and fish in their diet.

If you feel that you might be suffering from a potassium deficiency a simple blood test and examination will identify the problem. It is treated with a combination of diet and supplementation but these should only be taken under medical supervision to ensure the correct dosage is given and that there are no interactions with any medications.

If you are currently taking NSAIDs such as ibuprofen you should not take potassium supplements without medical advice. This applies to ACE inhibitors (elevated blood pressure), diuretics, Heparin (blood clots), Cyclosporine (anti-rejection drug) Trimethoprim (anti-biotic) and Beta Blockers (high blood pressure). All these drugs can increase the levels of potassium in your blood leading to potential health issues.

What Are the Best Food Sources for Potassium?
There is a wide variety of foods that you can include in your daily diet that will supply you with adequate amounts of potassium.

It is found in most fresh fruit and vegetables, many of which are on our superfoods list. Apricots, avocados, bananas, Brussel sprouts, melon, dates, figs, kiwi fruit, milk, nectarines, oranges, pears, peanuts, potatoes, prune juice, raisins, spinach, tomato and yoghurt. If you combine these foods with magnesium and calcium rich foods your body will adjust the balance of potassium it needs to keep your heart and kidneys healthy. These would include broccoli, cheese, milk, salmon, sardines, beans, halibut, nuts, oysters, seeds and whole grains.

Selenium

Selenium has a number of crucial functions within the body including playing a part in healthy growth and reproduction. It is also needed to keep some of your major organs healthy including the liver and the heart. More importantly recent research is suggesting that it may protect you against cancer. Part of its power comes from the ability to act as an antioxidant, clearing the body of free radicals, which are the unstable oxygen molecules that cause DNA damage to cells, leading to tumours. It works best in conjunction with a group of nutrients including vitamin E, vitamin C and Vitamin B3. Most of the success has been in the laboratory where selenium has broken down carcinogens and encouraged damaged cells to self-destruct before they become cancerous. It is hoped that the selenium in our daily diet also provides this affect.

The selenium works by activating an antioxidant enzyme called glutathione peroxidase. Apart from its possible affect on cancers, selenium also is essential for a healthy functioning immune system by stimulating the activity of white blood cells, the primary component of the immune system. Our immune system like any essential function within the body is likely to be tired and not working as efficiently as it should. Selenium is therefore an important part of our daily diet and for men in particularly it may be very important in the prevention and treatment of prostate cancer.

Selenium may not only a preventative but also could help survival rates for those patients who are already suffering from cancer. However, as with any naturally occurring nutrient it must only be supplemented in large doses under the supervision of a medical professional. The recommended daily dose is 55 mcg per day for adults but the usual supplement for preventative and therapeutic benefits is between 200 mcg and 400 mcg.

A normal diet should provide more than enough selenium to keep you healthy and you should be getting around 100 mcg of the mineral per day from your food. One of the main concerns for nutritionists is that the soil that nourishes the food that we eat may be loosing its selenium content along with a number of other essential minerals. When tests have been carried out on rheumatoid arthritis sufferers and heart patients, selenium is one of the minerals that's levels are depleted. Many of these people show indications of following a healthy diet including those foods that should contain adequate levels of selenium. Again we have to question the nutrient quality of the fresh food we are consuming or our ability to process that food. My inclination is to the deterioration of our growing areas.

Some of the health areas that selenium plays a role other than cancer are asthma, depression, skin problems, heart disease, infertility, and reduced thyroid function. Symptoms of deficiency are weakness or pain in muscles, changes in the colouring of hair and skin and whitening of the bottom of the fingernails.

There are some cases of toxicity from exposure to excessive selenium in our environment and from over supplementation. It is rare but symptoms of toxicity would be nausea, vomiting, hair loss, skin lesions and abnormalities in the bed of the fingernails. If these symptoms are present it is more usually environmental exposure through industrial or soil pollution. The foods that contain selenium usually have levels of around 30–50 mcg per serving except for Brazil nuts that contain 70–90 mcg per nut.

What Are the Best Food Sources for Selenium?

The best food sources of selenium are liver, fish such as halibut, cod, salmon and tuna. Mushrooms particularly shitake are a great source and very important if you are vegetarian. Brazil nuts are a great snack and taking one or two a couple of times a day will provide you with adequate amounts in addition to your other nutrient rich foods.

Sodium

Sodium is an essential macro-mineral that along with potassium helps to regulate the body's fluid balance. It is an electrolyte (cation), which is a positively electrically charged atom that performs essential tasks within each cell. Unlike other minerals, sodium or sodium chloride (table salt) has a very recognisable and almost addictive taste. It is very widely used in all processed foods and it is very easy to consume unhealthy amounts in our diet.

One of the main medical conditions associated with excessive sodium intake is very high blood pressure and heart disease so keeping a check on our intake is vitally important. This is one of the leading causes of premature death that can easily be prevented by making some small but significant changes to your lifestyle.

If you are trying to lose weight you may find that reducing your sodium intake will allow you to lose a great deal of water that has been retained in the cells due to the high level of salt in the blood.

Sodium deficiency is rare and in fact it is estimated that we are consuming at least 5 times the amount of sodium that we should be.

What Are the Current Recommendations for Sodium?

The current recommendation is under 2,400 mg of sodium per day, which is approximately one level teaspoon of table salt. If I give you some comparisons for processed foods versus fresh foods you will see how quickly you can take in far more than your body needs.

- Half a can of baked beans contains 504 mg of sodium – fresh contains 5 mg of sodium
- Half a can of mushrooms contains 400 mg of sodium – fresh contains 1 mg of sodium
- Half a can of tomatoes with spices is 600 mg of sodium-homemade would be 4 mg of sodium.
- 3 oz of salty bacon contains 1,197 mg of sodium – fresh pork chop 54 mg of sodium
- A chicken frozen dinner contains 2,500 mg of sodium – freshly prepared 50 mg of sodium.
- Packet of dry minestrone soup contains 6,400 mg – freshly prepared 100 mg.

Some other foods that we might eat on a regular basis have equally horrifying amounts of sodium including baked ham, 3 oz = 840 mg; French salad dressing, 2 tablespoons = 438 mg; half jar of Alfredo pasta sauce =1,080 mg; half can of chicken noodle soup = 1,160 mg.

How Can We Reduce the Salt in Our Diets?

By now you will have gathered that I am not keen on processed foods. Apart from the fact you have little or no idea exactly where the food has come from you certainly do not have full knowledge of the manufacturing processes or the number of people who have been involved in the finished product.

We now have labels on food and for the most part, although they seem to be written in stupidly small print (mainly because there are so many ingredients they have not got room on the jar) we can find out how much of a certain additive there is in any processed foods that we buy.

There are sodium reduced products on the market but be careful about the substitutes that have been use to produce this supposedly safe product. One of the most popular taste additives is MSG (monosodium glutamate) and that can sometimes be slipped in without you recognising it.

- Only eat canned soups, broths and stock cubes rarely unless you are sure they are sodium reduced or free.
- Avoid bacon and cured meats on a regular basis.
- Avoid salty snacks.
- Use salt free butter or olive oil.
- Check the sodium contents on any processed foods that you buy and choose the lower sodium brands. This applies to mineral water, which can have as much as 60 mg of sodium per 100 ml. That is 1200 mg per 2 litres bottle which easy to drink on a hot day.
- Make eating takeaways an exception not the rule.
- Use fresh fruit, vegetables, meat, fish and chicken products rather than canned or pre-prepared.
- Instant cereals, breakfast cereals, instant rice, pastas etc. usually have high levels of sodium.
- All sauces like ketchup are very high in sugar so only use a bare amount on the side of your plate rather than on your food.
- Always get sauces on the side when you are in a restaurant and use only the barest to give a taste to your food.

- If you are cooking for the family use a pot of salt containing 1/2 level teaspoon of salt for each family member. Remember that if you all have had breakfast cereal that you will have already consumed sodium during the day so ½ teaspoon per person for cooking will help to keep the total levels down.
- Be aware of aliases in the form of monosodium glutamate, sodium nitrate, sodium saccharin, baking soda (sodium bicarbonate) and sodium benzoate.

Zinc

Zinc has been called 'the healing mineral'. There is evidence to suggest that wounds heal faster when the body has sufficient zinc in reserve and a patient who has a healthy diet including foods containing zinc may find that recovery from operations is speeded up. In some cases additional supplementation is recommended, particularly in a person who has not got a healthy diet.

Zinc is also plays a major role in respiratory infections, burns and skin conditions and certainly has shown that if used in the form of lozenges at the start of a cold, it can alleviate some of the symptoms.

Like Vitamin C, Zinc is a component of more than 300 enzymes needed to repair wounds, maintain fertility in adults and growth in children. It helps synthesise protein, helps cells reproduce, protects vision, boosts immunity and acts as an antioxidant, protecting us from free radical damage.

The primary areas of health that the mineral is most effectively used are for acne, common cold, Down's syndrome, infertility, night blindness and wound healing. It is also used therapeutically in certain cases of anaemia, anorexia nervosa, birth defect prevention, celiac disease, cold sores, Crohn's disease, Diabetes, mouth and gum disorders, liver disease, and peptic ulcers. This list is only a partial representation of the areas of health that Zinc is involved in and including it in your daily diet is very important.

One of the areas that I have used zinc as part of a diet programme is for men in their mid 40's onwards. Prostate problems such as enlargement or even cancer are quite common in that age group and zinc is one of the minerals that may help prevent future problems. In this case a handful of pumpkinseeds twice a day provides a healthy dose of zinc as well as other nutrients.

How Would We Know If We Were Deficient in Zinc?

A major deficiency is unlikely in the western world. In under developed countries children who are deficient suffer from stunted growth, weight loss, gastrointestinal problems and pneumonia.

In our environment there is some evidence that if there is a poor diet prior to and during pregnancy that zinc will be deficient that could lead to birth defects and illness in the mother. Drinking alcohol to excess can result in liver damage, particularly liver cirrhosis and there appears to be a link to zinc deficiency.

An interesting line of research is in the management of Down's syndrome. Children born with this syndrome are commonly deficient in Zinc and are treated with a supplement and diet and this helps boost their immunity and thyroid function, which is suppressed due to the condition.

The most common age group for deficiency is the elderly whose digestive systems, along with many other operational activities has slowed down and is complicated by a decrease in appetite and the resultant lack of food and nourishment. If kidney disease is also present the effects the deficiency could be worsened.

Are There Any Dangers if You Include Zinc in Your Diet?

Including zinc in your everyday diet is unlikely to cause problems. If you are deficient a supplement containing 15 mg per day is sufficient unless your doctor advises higher doses for certain illnesses.

There is evidence to suggest that once you start taking in excess of 300 mg per day in supplements you could impair immune system function rather than boosting it.

Some people find that zinc lozenges that are taken at the start of a cold leave a metallic taste in them mouth and some experience gastrointestinal problems but it is usually due to taking more than the recommended dosage, in excess of 150 mg. This is one of those cases where less may be more.

The best food sources for zinc are: seafood particularly oysters, pumpkinseeds, sesame seeds, wheat germ, egg yolks, black-eyed peas and tofu.

Summary

- You now have some of the basic ingredients necessary to provide your body with the correctly balanced mix of nutrients. In addition to this, the growing, live food that you eat is protected by its own defence systems and these are passed to you when you consume them.
- Brightly coloured foods contain antioxidants, flavanoids and other substances that offer not only the plant protection but the end user. As you will see from the next section food is not just about taste but also about the prevention and healing of illnesses.

Part Three –
Food & Exercise

Foods to Give You the Right Fuel Mix!

The word 'Superfood' is now being hugely overused. When I first used the term it was to illustrate that a particular food was especially packed with the nutrients that are considered vital for good health.

I encourage you to eat as many varieties of fresh fruit and vegetables with lean protein and whole grains to get as many of the nutrients as possible. All fresh foods that are prepared naturally have their health benefits and the foods that follow are simply a cross section to illustrate how one individual food can offer so much protection to your body and health.

You will hear academics claim that the ancient skills of healing with herbs and certain foods are mumbo jumbo. They are of course entitled to their learned opinion and I myself have little time for unsubstantiated miracle cures.

However, in my own experience over the years I have found that diet is fundamental to a long and healthy life and also to a fit and energetic old age.

If you look at sprightly 80 and 90 year olds with all their marbles it is no surprise to find that most have remained active, maintained their appetite for life and food and usually eaten a mainly natural diet. I am not sure that the 80 and 90 year olds of fifty years ahead will be in the same state of health. They may well be kept alive by medication and modern science rather than diet and having seen some elderly people on this regime I can tell you the quality of life is not as good as for those who have enjoyed a healthy lifestyle.

Today most foods are available all year round but a word of caution. Foods that come from abroad may not have ripened on the plant and may have been forced as well as coloured to provide you with what you think that vegetable or fruit should look like.

Try whenever possible to buy locally grown produce and if you are lucky enough to live near a farm shop then you will find it cheaper and probably healthier to buy your fresh produce there. Obviously some of the more exotic produce will have to be bought from the supermarket and I have found that taste is usually the give away. An avocado that is naturally ripened has a rich buttery taste and is slightly soft. Oranges travel fairly well but should be juicy and slightly sweet. Over time you will get the idea and use your taste buds as a test for whether a fruit or vegetable is as it should be.

The aim of this section is to get you to look at food in a different way. Learning a little bit about its history and its evolution may give you a respect for it and also a taste for it.

We tend to take the food that we eat for granted. For many men a plate is put in front of them by first their mother and then their partner. For those who fend for themselves, cooking may not fit into the busy work and social part of their lives. Food can take hours to prepare and then minutes to eat and it is not 'thoughtful' eating. It is taking the essential fuel we need to survive for granted without appreciating its value.

I can't write about all foods in this section as the book would be a trilogy but I hope that these particular favourites of mine will give you a flavour of what is available to you that are tasty, healthy and nutrient packed.

Carbohydrates

We looked at carbohydrates in relation to sugars in an earlier chapter but it is important to understand this complex fuel as it is vital that our body receives adequate amounts so that we are provided with the energy we need to live.

It used to be that the recommendation was to fill up on your 'carbs' then came the Atkin's diet and we were told not to eat them at all and in the end it becomes all too confusing.

Like any food there are good and bad carbohydrates. Some you can eat all your life without them harming you and others can lead to heart disease or diabetes.

The simple rule is 'if it is white, don't eat it'. So we are talking about white bread and flour products, most white rice (Basmati is a useful exception as it does act in a similar way to brown rice), cakes, biscuits and cookies, pastries and sugary products such as sweets, chocolates and fizzy drinks.

The carbohydrates you need to include are the whole grains in bread and pasta, beans, fruits and vegetables.

You cannot simply remove a food group and expect your body to function efficiently. Our bodies are over 100,000 years old and have managed quite successfully to evolve to changing conditions over the centuries but unfortunately modern life has surpassed itself with its ability to process the hell out of most things natural.

Carbohydrates are either simple which includes the sugars such as fruit (fructose) corn (dextrose or glucose) and table (sucrose). Complex sugars on the other hand are made up of three or four sugar molecules in a chain.

The body breaks down all carbohydrates in the same way to the lowest common denominator which is one single sugar molecule as this is the only size that can pass into the bloodstream. The body also needs to provide energy to the cells so it converts the most easily digestible carbohydrate into glucose or blood sugar.

When your blood sugar rises, cells in the pancreas produces the hormone insulin which signals the cells to absorb the blood sugar to use immediately for energy or to store for later use. As the blood sugar is absorbed into the cells the levels naturally drop in the blood and the pancreas then switches over to another function which is to produce glucagon. This release of glucagon is a signal to the liver where blood sugar is stored to release more into the system ensuring that the body is provided with energy on a consistent level.

Sometimes this complex communication system fails as a result of Type 1 diabetes where enough insulin is not produced or Type 2 diabetes where the cells do not respond when told to absorb blood sugar. This leads to a condition called insulin resistance which enables sugar levels and insulin levels to stay too high following food consumption.

You will have seen in the section on Diabetes that Type 2 is very definitely linked to other lifestyle conditions such as obesity, high blood pressure and elevated cholesterol.

Most people by now have heard of the Glycemic Index in relation to carbohydrates. What the body requires is a slow steady release of blood sugar over an extended period rather than several quick and high spikes in levels which result in the miscommunication we talked about above.

White carbohydrates are the culprits for this kind of release and the complex or whole grain carbohydrates are the good guys.

You will find also that alleged whole grains that have been heavily processed might also have the same affect as the white carbohydrates so be aware that eating supposed healthy whole grain cakes, biscuits and bread may not be good for you.

As I keep reinforcing – look at the labels and just see how many preservatives and additives including colourants and sugars are in the whole grain bread on the shelf.

Ideally, make it yourself – there are a number of electronic bread makers around these days that only require you to put in the ingredients. At the very least see if your grocery shop or health food shop offer a selection of more naturally produced bread.

You also need carbohydrates that have fibre. In the section below you will see how important this is to your weight and your health and fibre is not left in the white processed carbohydrates.

Carbohydrates are also available in fruit and vegetables and whilst there is an argument to reduce (not remove) the amount of starchy carbohydrates from our diet as we get older and perhaps less active, there is absolutely no excuse to remove the essential fruits and vegetables that contain carbohydrates from our diet.

Begin the day with slow releasing carbohydrates and take another portion in at lunchtime. After that I find it useful to rely on fruit and vegetables to provide the higher percentage of carbohydrates except for the occasional rice cake for example as a snack.

Apart from energy and fibre you will see from the break down of the individual carbohydrates below, that there is also a wealth of nutrients present that are usually stripped out completely in processing.

Carbohydrates To Include in Your Diet

Beans

Mention the fact that you are an ardent bean lover and people automatically give you a wide berth. Unfortunately this very nutritious food group has developed a rather anti-social reputation over the years but prepared and cooked correctly beans can overcome their wind producing properties.

History of the Bean

There is evidence going back nearly 12,000 years that peas were part of the staple diet in certain cultures and certainly natives of Peru and Mexico were cultivating beans as a crop 9,000 years ago. It is likely that they were one of the first crops to be planted when man ceased to be nomadic and settled into communities.

There are many types of bean used as a staple food in different cultures around the world including Black beans, Chickpeas, Kidney Beans, Navy Beans and Soybeans. In Asia where consumption of soybean products is very high it is regarded as one of the best preventative medicines that you can eat.

What Are the Main Health Benefits of Beans?

For anyone suffering high cholesterol levels, blood pressure, heart disease, constipation, irritable bowel syndrome, Diverticulitis, colon cancer, diabetes or iron deficiency, beans are definitely on the healthy foods list. One of the main health benefits of eating beans is their high fibre content.

Although fibre is not exactly up there on everyone's favourite foods list it is extremely important to our overall health. Fibre is carbohydrate that cannot be digested and there are two types, water-soluble and water insoluble. Primarily water-soluble fibre comes from oatmeal, oat bran, nuts and seeds, fruit and legumes that include peas, lentils and beans. The insoluble fibre is mainly found in whole grains, wheat bran, seeds, root vegetables, cucumbers, courgettes, celery and tomatoes.

Fibre acts like a vacuum cleaner, travelling through the bloodstream and intestines collecting cholesterol plaque, toxins, waste products from normal bodily functions and anything else that should not be there.

Provided you do not pile high fat sauces and butter onto this group of foods they can be a very healthy aid to weight loss as fibre has no calories and the foods containing it are generally low in fat and high in nutrients.

What Else Is in Beans That Is Healthy?

Beans are packed with nutrients as well as fibre including Vitamin B1 (thiamin) copper, folate, iron, magnesium, manganese, phosphorus and tryptophan. The combination of nutrients will help boost your immune system, balance blood sugar levels, lower your risk of heart disease and help protect you against cancer.

Vitamin B1 (thiamin) is essential in the metabolism of carbohydrates and for a healthy nervous system. Every cell in the body requires this vitamin to form the fuel the body runs on, ATP (Adenosine Triphosphate).

Copper is an essential trace mineral needed to absorb and utilise iron and also assist in the production of collagen.

Folate is a B vitamin essential for cell replication and growth. It is needed for our nervous system and heart health as folate helps lower homocysteine levels in the blood, a leading contributory factor in heart disease.

Magnesium is an essential mineral needed for bone, protein and fatty acid formation, forming new cells, activating the B vitamins, relaxing muscles, clotting blood and forming ATP. The secretion and action of insulin also needs magnesium as does the correct balance of calcium in the body.

Iron is an integral part of the oxygen-carrying haemoglobin in the blood, which is why a deficiency can cause fatigue and ill health.

Manganese boosts energy and the immune system and molybdenum another trace mineral helps detox the body of sulphites a commonly used preservative in processed food and one that many people have sensitivity to.

Tryptophan is an amino acid that is critical in the manufacture of serotonin a neurotransmitter that affects our mental wellbeing.

Preparing Beans to Avoid the Wind Factor

If you are not used to fibre then you need to introduce it into your diet over a period of days. This guideline applies to eating beans as people who eat them regularly seem to have less of a problem. There are a number of helpful tips to ensure that you receive all of the benefits and none of the more anti-social side effects.

Soak your dried beans for at least 6 hours before cooking. Change the water several times.

Put the beans in a large pot and cover with cold unsalted water usually 3 to 6 times the amount of beans. Bring to the boil and reduce to a simmer. Drain the beans after 30 minutes and replace the water. Bring back to the boil and then simmer.

Skim off any foam that rises to the surface of the water.

When the beans have softened add some salt, as this will bring out their flavour. If you add salt at the beginning of cooking it can make the beans tougher. If you are on a low sodium diet then be careful about how much salt you add, or use an alternative.

When the beans are cooked you can prepare in a number of ways. Include in brown rice dishes; stir-fry with a little olive oil, seasonings and favourite spices.

A lovely way to eat beans is in a casserole with tomatoes, onions, garlic, olive oil, carrots, potatoes, celery and vegetable stock.

Make your own baked beans with homemade tomato sauce and serve on jacket potatoes or on toast.

You can blend with other ingredients and make hamburgers, meatloaves and pates.

Brown Rice

It is important to remove toxins from the body safely and gently. Brown rice is not only full of nutrients that will help support your liver and your body during this process but it also provides essential fibre.

As the body releases waste and toxins from the cells and tissues it will pass through to the intestines. There are some normal side effects that might occur as this takes place but if you include fibre, particularly brown rice the toxins will be removed quickly and efficiently.

What Is so Special About Brown Rice?

Brown rice will contain more nutrients than white rice as it loses only the outer layer of the grain called the hull. During the process that turns brown rice to white rice it loses 67% of its vitamin B3 (niacin) 80% of B1, 90% of B6 – half of its manganese and phosphorus, 60% of its iron and all the dietary fibre and essential fatty acids. Do you realise that to make white rice acceptable as a food it has to be artificially enriched with B1 B3 and iron? It is amazing the difference that processing a food can have on its nutritional content.

Brown rice is a very rich source of manganese – essential for blood health. It is also necessary for bone health and for its antioxidant capabilities in preventing damage to cells, particularly blood cells.

Brown rice is rich in fibre, which cleans the system of toxins and harmful deposits in the blood so helps keep your cholesterol down. Like oats it tends to release its energy slowly so maintaining stable blood sugar levels. The fibre is insoluble which means that it works through your system efficiently. This prevents some organs from getting into an overload situation like the liver and the bile duct – a speedy process through the system ensures that the bile duct does not secrete too much bile which can lead to gallstones.

Brown rice is high in selenium which is essential for our immune systems and thyroid function – also to help prevent cancer as it encourages healthy DNA repair in the cells.

Magnesium is present in high quantities and this is associated with a number of systemic problems such as asthma – high blood pressure – migraine headaches and reducing the risk of heart attacks and strokes. Magnesium does this because it helps to regulate nerve and muscle tone by balancing the action of calcium. You will see that very often calcium supplements are teamed with magnesium.

Calcium tends to rush around frantically and needs magnesium to curb its enthusiasm. For example if allowed to, calcium will overwhelm the nerve cells in the muscles and get them all wound up and over activated. This causes the muscle to overwork and wear out faster. This can happen if you have insufficient magnesium in your diet. Another reason that magnesium is so important is for bone health and about two thirds of the magnesium is found in the bones of the human body. The rest is stored for when needed. Brown rice provides nearly a quarter of your daily requirement in one serving.

The human body is over 100,000 years old. In that time the body has developed an incredible defence mechanism called the survival instinct. In some cases it is miraculous. It is only in recent centuries that we have begun to refine our grains. Our bodies spent the first 99,990 years eating whole-grains including rice. Wheat only came along about 10,000 years ago. So our bodies evolved a very precise dietary support system that provided it with everything it needed to survive and be the fittest. It was essential for the survival of mankind that only the fittest made it through. This ensured that each generation was stronger.

If you go back to what I was saying about the loss of nutrients in the processing of brown rice to white rice you can perhaps understand why we are now facing the sort of medical problems that we are.

Oats

Of all the grains – oats are one of the most versatile – from porridge to sugar free muesli and also baked in bread and biscuits. You can also buy an oat drink, which is very like milk, and you can use this as an alternative to dairy.

Their Latin name is Avena Sativa and if you go into a health food shop you will find quite a few medicinal products labelled this way.

When oats are harvested they are cleaned and then roasted which is what gives them their flavour. Their bran and their germ are not affected by this process which means that they are a wholegrain and have a high concentration of nutrients.

Oats are particularly high in Manganese, which is a very important anti-oxidant in cell health and the prevention of anaemia. It also has Selenium, Tryptophan (a precursor or project manager for Serotonin which we will talk about in a minute) Phosphorus, Vitamin B1, Magnesium and some protein.

Oats contain a special fibre called beta-glucan – this particular fibre is very good for lowering cholesterol and can help prevent blood disorders that are prone to high cholesterol, particularly something like diabetes. Therefore this is great for preventing heart disease and strokes as the plaque in your bloodstream will not be blocking the arteries and allowing free flow of oxygenated blood. It is what is called a low glycemic food. This is good because instead to sending your blood sugars very high and then dropping them like a stone a little while later as many carbohydrates can do – oats are a slow releasing fuel that means that your sugar levels are taken to a moderate level. This provides you with energy and then maintains those levels over a longer period of time.

Which is why porridge will give you more energy for longer.

Apart from helping maintain stable blood sugar levels – the fibre in oats has also been shown to be anti-bacterial and helps your immune system with wound healing.

I mentioned selenium, which is another great anti-oxidant – primarily in the repair of the DNA of cells especially in the colon. It also works with vitamin C in the lungs and if you are an asthma sufferer you may find that a bowl of oatmeal for breakfast will help your condition.

Oats are also important for sufferers from wheat intolerances as there seems to be either a smaller amount of gluten or its affects are less because of the oats makeup.

What Is Serotonin?

Tryptophan is an amino acid, which is associated with an increase in serotonin levels in the brain. Higher serotonin levels have a calming affect and you will often see that natural sleeping products contain tryptophan to stimulate both serotonin and melatonin another calming hormone. Serotonin can not be passed to the brain via oral supplements – it cannot be synthesised or manufactured. However tryptophan is a precursor or project manager that increases the production of serotonin. Serotonin plays a vital role in how we feel – depression and stress are some of the areas that this hormone governs. This is why it is often called the 'feel good hormone' and is what we get after eating chocolate. Eating oats not only makes us feel better throughout the day it is one of the only grains that raises our serotonin levels and maintains them longer in the day. Although tryptophan also stimulates an increase in melatonin – that hormone cannot be activated before night as it is regulated by light – therefore eating oats is not going to make you sleepy but taking an hot oat drink at night might help you sleep.

So, to summarise – oats provide you with fibre and anti-oxidants and are easily tolerable. They help put you into a good mood and feel better longer throughout the day. They have been shown to help prevent high cholesterol, diabetes, heart disease and cancers.

The Potato

The potato is one of the carbohydrates that have fallen out of favour in recent years with the advent of the Low Carbohydrate diet. By removing this vegetable completely from the diet the body will be missing out on many nutrients that it depends upon to be healthy. Having said that, it is a starchy vegetable and if you are already a couch potato it needs to be included as part of your daily diet within the recommendations of your calorie requirements. Frying in the form of chips or as roast potatoes adds large amounts of fats, so preparation is key.

There are some legends regarding the introduction of the potato into Ireland around 1600. Some authorities believe that Sir Frances Drake brought specimens back from the West Indies and handed some over to Sir Walter Raleigh who cultivated them on his farm in Ireland. I prefer the far more quirky explanation that potatoes were washed up on the shore after the Armada was sunk and with typical Irish ingenuity were transformed into a national treasure and the basis of a traditional alcoholic beverage.

This humble root vegetable has travelled thousands of miles to adorn our dinner plates and there is archaeological evidence that they were first cultivated in Peru around 4500 years ago although wild potatoes had been eaten as early as 10,000 years ago. Wheat and corn could not survive the cold of the mountains in the same way as the potato and the Inca cultures actually developed frost-resistant varieties and a technique to freeze dry the mature root, providing flour that could be stored for a number of years. As in Ireland in the 1800's the potato became the staple food for South American's living at high altitudes and they even produced alcohol in the form of a beer called chicha.

Despite its recent disfavour with the diet industry, in actual fact calorie wise the potato has far less than rice, pasta and bread and provided it is not laden with cheese and butter, is a highly nutritious, low fat and healthy accompaniment to any meal.

There are over 100 different cultivated potatoes available around the world and some of the more familiar to us are the King Edward, Maris Piper, Kerr's Pink and Rooster varieties. Some older varieties were reflective of the time they were cultivated, such as Irish Peace.

What Are the Health Benefits of the Potato?

There is a very good reason why the potato has been regarded as a staple food in so many cultures. When nothing else will grow and conditions are tough the potato will thrive and provide many essential nutrients the body needs to survive.

Provided you do not eat a pound of fat with your potatoes, including them as part of your diet may prevent a number of potentially serious illnesses. Research into elevated cholesterol levels, high blood pressure, heart disease, Alzheimer's disease, poor immune system function, cancer and hormonal imbalance show that the properties in the potato could well help prevent these conditions from developing in the first place. If you need to lose weight, eating potatoes will provide you with a great many nutrients and energy without adding excess calories or fats to your daily diet.

Despite being around for thousands of years this vegetable still holds surprises and recently scientists have isolated kukoamines in potatoes, which have only been previously found in some Chinese herbal remedies. The main property of this chemical is its ability to reduce blood pressure levels. As elevated blood pressure is becoming increasingly more common for both men and women, eating potatoes regularly in the diet could be very beneficial.

Potatoes are also high in Vitamin C, B6, Copper, Potassium, manganese and fibre. They also contain phytonutrients called flavanoids and carotenoids that are extremely important anti-oxidants.

Most of us are familiar with the health benefits of Vitamin C especially in relation to our immune system, but this vitamin also protects the harmful cholesterol LDL from oxidative damage, which leads to plaque forming and blocking our arteries. The potato also contains Vitamin B6 which is involved in nearly every major process in the body. Copper which is needed for the ATP, the fuel we run on, Potassium which creates the perfect working environment in and around each cell and Manganese needed for healthy skin, bone and cartilage as well as glucose intolerance.

It is important that you eat the skin of the potato as this contains a concentrated source of fibre, which our bodies need to remove waste and toxins efficiently. If you buy pre-washed potatoes you will need to clean before eating, as the potato will have become susceptible to fungus and bacterial contamination. Scrub the potato under running water and remove any eyes or bruises before cooking. You can boil, bake, dry roast, mash and dice potatoes. If you want to mash or roast with a little fat, use olive oil and herbs rather than butter or margarine.

Next time you pass the display of potatoes in a supermarket don't think "fattening," think "mashed with a little olive oil and garlic or roasted with rosemary and Mediterranean vegetables with a little lamb on the side"

Fruits

Apricot

The apricot season opens at the beginning of May and goes through to the end of August or early September, which gives us five months to enjoy this highly nutritious and healing food.

First though a little history about this luscious golden yellow fruit. In China over 4000 years ago a bride will have not only had something borrowed and something blue but would have also been nibbling on an apricot. It was prized for its ability to increase fertility, which is not surprising, as it is high in nutrients necessary for the production of sex hormones.

The Latin name for the apricot is "praecocia" which means precocious or early ripening. It is part of the rose family and is a cousin to the peach, plum, cherry and the almond. In China it first grew wild in the mountains before being introduced to Arab traders who took it with them along the trade routes to Babylon and Persia where they were called the "eggs of the sun". Over the following centuries the fruit continued its travels reaching Greece where the juice was known as "nectar of the Gods, then onto Spain, Mexico and North America. It is now cultivated in all warm climates around the world and used as a sweet and savoury addition to a healthy diet.

What Are the Benefits of the Apricot?

As with any fresh fruit the apricot is packed with fibre and nutrients including Vitamin A, Vitamin C, Vitamins B1, B2, B6, Vitamin E, Potassium and Iron. Of particular interest from a therapeutic viewpoint are its high levels of carotenoids.

Carotenoids are responsible for the wonderfully rich reds, oranges and yellow colouring of plant leaves, fruits, flowers and some birds, insects and fish such as salmon. There are around

600 carotenoids that occur naturally and the apricot has two in particular that benefit us, Beta-carotene and lycopene.

Beta-carotene is converted into Vitamin A in the body. Vitamin A is essential for healthy sight especially at night. As with any part of the body the sensitive components of the eye are as vulnerable to oxidative damage as any other and Vitamin A deficiency has been linked to degenerative eye disease in many research programmes. It has also shown that eating just three portions a day of yellow and orange fruit and vegetables such as apricots and carrots would lower the risk of poor eyesight as we age.

As an anti-oxidant, beta-carotene protects the LDL or harmful cholesterol from free radical damage that can cause plaque to form in the arteries. A build up of plaque can lead to both heart disease and a higher risk of stroke.

Lycopene is usually associated with bright red fruits such as tomatoes but it is also present in apricots. As well as helping protect the eyes from degenerative disease, lycopene is associated with a reduction in damage to LDL cholesterol and a much lower risk of developing a number of cancers including bladder, breast, cervix, prostate and skin.

There has been considerable interest in the medicinal properties of the apricot kernel for the last 40 years. There have been some controversial claims made about cancer curing abilities that has not been well received by the medical profession or pharmaceutical companies. Hopefully ongoing research will prove that this is a natural alternative to the highly invasive treatments currently available such as chemotherapy and radiation therapy. Modern scientists are not the first researchers in history to explore the possibilities of the apricot kernel.

What Are the Medicinal Uses of Apricots?

In ancient China over 4,000 years ago, healers used a medicine made from the kernels to prolong life. Additionally the oils from the kernels were used as a sedative, muscle relaxant, in wound healing and as an anti-parasitic.

The apricot's fibre makes it a gentle laxative; aids weight loss and reduces cholesterol in the blood. Its alkaline properties aid digestion if eaten before a meal and due to the high content of iron it is excellent for anyone suffering from anaemia. Apricots also contain a small but essential amount of copper, which may increase the production of haemoglobin in the blood providing more oxygen and therefore energy for the body.

Over the centuries the juice of apricots mixed with honey has been used to treat fevers and the juice from the leaves appears to reduce the inflammation caused by eczema and sunburn.

So this small fruit has a large reputation and certainly in the fight against the most common modern diseases such as elevated cholesterol, heart disease and cancers it would definitely be worth including in your diet on a daily basis.

Buying Apricots

Apricots are best eaten when still a little firm. If they are not fully ripe when you buy them keep them in a fruit bowl for two to three days and then store in paper or plastic bag in the fridge for up to three days.

Apart from eating them fresh you can use them in cooking by stewing, grilling, baking or roasting and they are delicious as an accompaniment to meat and poultry dishes or in desserts. As a pre dinner snack they are delicious halved and stuffed with a cream cheese and chopped nuts. For a main course serve in a fresh spinach and walnut salad with roast salmon.

If you want to use dried apricots out of season then do buy guaranteed sulphite free brands as there are many people who react to this preservative. Asthma sufferers in particular should avoid any food containing sulphites including inexpensive wine, baked goods, soup mixes, jams, snacks and most dried fruit.

Avocado

If ever there was a food to include in your daily diet, it is the Avocado and it has been on my list of 'superfoods' for some years now.

Many people mistakenly believe that this fruit is fattening and should be avoided if they are to lose weight. On the contrary, the benefits of eating avocados far outweigh its slightly elevated fat content.

What Is the History of the Avocado?

Avocados are native to Central and South America and have been cultivated in these regions for over 8000 years. The Aztecs called the fruit 'ahuacati' or testicle because of its shape; the Spanish

Conquistadors were unable to pronounce this word correctly and adapted it to agaucate. The Aztecs regarded the avocado a powerful aphrodisiac and in later centuries producers had to counteract this reputation so that moral and upstanding citizens would buy the fruit.

Since the 16th century, when the Spanish first wrote about the avocado its consumption has spread throughout the world. In fact those early written accounts may well have utilised a unique property of the avocado. The Spanish discovered that if you open the kernel and expose the milky white liquid to air it turns to reddish brown or black and could be used as ink. Following its discovery in South America, travellers next encountered it in the West Indies and George Washington wrote in 1751 that 'agovago pears' were abundant and popular in Barbados.

What Makes the Avocado so Special?

Avocados are a wonderful source of Essential Fatty Acids which we covered in the chapter on nutrients.

EFAs are so important because they support our cardiovascular, reproductive, immune and nervous systems. We need these fats to manufacture and repair cells, maintain hormone levels and expel waste from the body. They are part of the process that regulates blood pressure, blood clotting, fertility, conception and help regulate inflammation and stimulate the body to fight infection.

The avocado has one of these EFA's in abundance, the non-essential Oleic acid (Omega 9) and there is growing evidence that it may help to lower cholesterol by decreasing LDL (low-density lipoprotein) unhealthy cholesterol but at the same time raising HDL (high density lipoprotein) or healthy cholesterol.

Oleic acid is also emerging as a regulator of blood sugar levels and a possible protection against breast and prostate cancer, so including a half of an avocado in your diet every day may well protect you from the harmful and long term affects of a number of diseases.

What About the Other Nutrients in Avocados?

The avocado is packed with nutrients including Folate, B vitamins, Vitamin C, E and K as well as potassium, magnesium, copper, phosphorus, zinc and manganese.

It also contains Lutein which is a carotenoid, a natural pigment found in dark green vegetables. Lutein is an important antioxidant particular for our eyesight as it reduces the level of free radical damage to the eyes and skin from excessive exposure to the blue light from sunlight and indoor lighting.

Lutein has been associated with reduced risk of prostate cancer, however in tests it shows that obtaining it from a source such as the avocado is more effective than taking lutein as a lone supplement. It is thought that the body uses the combinations of carotenoids and also the Vitamin E content in the fruit to help prevent cancerous cell growth and reproduction.

Vitamin K is essential for synthesising the liver protein that controls blood clotting. It is also involved in bone formation and repair and therefore could reduce the risk or severity of osteoporosis.

Avocados have a healthy potassium content, the mineral that helps regulate blood pressure and possibly reduces the risk of strokes. Potassium also ensures that the body has the correct water balance and that plays an important part in the response of nerves to stimulation and in the contraction of muscles.

Vitamin E is a powerful antioxidant that is associated with a healthy heart. It prevents the oxidation of LDL cholesterol preventing blocked arteries; it acts as an anticoagulant, preventing blood clots leading to thrombosis. It reduces inflammation and it also appears to affect a key enzyme in the liver, which regulates the synthesis of cholesterol in the first place.

For a pregnant woman eating avocados will provide folic acid (folate) that is needed for the healthy cell and tissue development of a foetus. It will help also protect the baby against birth defects in the early stages of pregnancy and the vitamin B6 in the fruit has been shown to help relieve morning sickness.

How to Eat Avocados

Avocados should be ripe and you can test for this by cradling the avocado gently in your hand and gently squeezing the fruit. It should yield but still be firm. If it is ripe then use the flesh chopped on salads or halve the avocado and fill with seafood or roasted vegetables. It you have a very ripe avocado then mash with a little lemon juice and use as a spread or to make guacamole.

Bananas

Over the years I have heard many clients tell me that they do not eat bananas because they are fattening. This is from some people, myself included, who have thought nothing of consuming a 1000-calorie bar of chocolate or tub of ice cream in one sitting. I hope by the time you have read this section you will be converted to banana power and including them in your diet several times a week.

Originally the banana came from Malaysia and from there they were taken by visitors back to India in the 6th century BC. Alexander the Great loved eating bananas on his campaign through India and he is allegedly the person who introduced this fruit to the Western world. There is some evidence that they were grown in the southern parts of China but they were considered an exotic fruit that was only fit for royal consumption.

Unfortunately, ivory and slaves were part of a thriving business for Arabic traders as far back as 1500 years ago. More humane was the trade in the abundant crop of bananas that spread the word about the fruit throughout the islands of Africa. In turn in the 15th century, Portuguese sailors who landed on these Islands, took the rootstock of the banana tree back to the Canary Islands were the plantations in the Western world were established. From here the banana spread to every available and suitable growing site.

The word banana comes from the Arabic word banan for finger, as the original fruit were small and looked like a man's finger.

It was the 19th century before the Banana reached the United States and the UK and since then it has become one of our favourite fruits.

There are over 300 varieties of bananas available around the world and the annual crop output is over 90 million tons per year. In the developing world the banana is the fourth most important staple food due to its high nutritional content. India is the top producer with over 20% of the world's bananas but countries in Latin American countries come second.

What Is in the Banana That Makes It so Special as a Superfood?

The banana is one of those fruits that is suitable to be eaten by everyone of any age. It is very easy to digest, rarely causes an allergy and contains natural sugars that are easily absorbed into the bloodstream. It is packed with nutrients including protein comprising three essential amino acids and made into a milkshake it provides a highly nutritious meal in a glass.

Even athletes can tap into its power by eating 30 minutes before a workout as the combination of carbohydrates, B vitamins (needed to metabolise carbohydrates quickly) and sugars provide lots of additional energy.

One of the most useful nutrients in a banana is potassium and one of the main reasons why including this fruit daily can ensure your body is working at optimum efficiency.

The banana also contains Vitamin A, B1, B2, B3, B6, Folate, Vitamin C, Calcium, Magnesium with trace amounts of Iron and Zinc.

Finally the banana contains a decent amount of fibre which is essential for your general health. It reduces cholesterol levels, improves blood sugar control and lowers your risk of heart attacks.

How Do You Buy the Best Bananas and Store Them?

You can buy yellow bananas all year round and most other varieties are available in major supermarkets. There is obviously more choice of variety closest to the sources in the Spanish, Philippine and Thai markets where you could find red bananas, plantains and sometimes ladies fingers.

Bananas should be slightly green, firm and without any bruises on their skin. If they have a grey tint and look dull they have been refrigerated too long. Plantains used for cooking have a little more flexibility but are easier to use when slightly more ripe.

Do not store unripe bananas in the fridge, as they will not ripen properly at lower temperatures. Once a banana is ripe you can then refrigerate for up to 10 days although their skins will turn black. Yellow/green bananas need about 2 days to ripen at room temperature and will not taste good until that process is completed. If you have too many bananas and they ripen too quickly, cut into chunks and wrap them in cling film. Put in the freezer and use in drinks, sauces or in baking.

You can eat a banana at any time of day, on breakfast cereal, mashed on toast, cut up in custard on in fruit and vegetable salads. They are great in pancakes, muffins, bread, milkshakes and mixed with fresh yoghurt.

They are great for taking out on a day trip and you can even include them in your favourite cocktail.

Not only is the banana packed with nutrients but it is also a definite winner in the therapeutic arena. The fruit has been around for at least a couple of thousand years and many cultures have used the banana in their fight against illness.

The banana has many talents including keeping your bowels healthy, reducing your risk or heart disease and strokes, protecting you from ulcers, improving blood pressure, boosting your energy and your mood and help you reduce water retention.

More specifically the banana is a medicine cabinet in its own right. If we look at the diverse diseases and conditions that it is connected to you will realise how important it is in your diet.

- Anaemia is the result of a lack of haemoglobin the oxygen-carrying agent in red blood cells. Iron is essential in the manufacture of this haemoglobin in the bone marrow and bananas are high in this mineral.
- High blood pressure and stress related conditions effect many people and not just as they age. More and more children and young adults are showing signs of following a poor diet, high in junk food and low in natural fresh produce. Junk food is high in salt, which in the form of sodium and in excess causes elevated blood pressure.

The potassium in bananas helps lower blood pressure by dilating blood vessels, enhancing he excretion of water and sodium from the body and suppressing the hormones that cause elevations in blood pressure.

Potassium helps normalise the heartbeat, sends oxygen to the brain and regulates water balance. When we are stressed our metabolic rate increases, reducing our potassium levels and by eating a banana we can help re-balance all these symptoms in one snack.

- Depression and nervous conditions can be helped by eating bananas as they contain tryptophan, a protein that converts into serotonin. Serotonin is a chemical in the brain that makes you relax and improves your mood. The B vitamins in the fruit are also essential for a healthy central nervous system.
- Heartburn is eased by eating a banana due to its antacid

effect, and it has the added benefit of not causing stomach problems when used long term.

- Ulcers in the stomach are very delicate and the banana is one of the few foods that can be eaten raw without causing any further distress or inflammation to the ulcer site. It also reduces over acidity and the irritation this causes to the lining of the stomach.
- PMS is dreadful not just for the woman concerned but usually for the family around her. Eating a banana with its B6 not only helps alleviate the stress symptoms but also works to regulate the hormones causing the problem.
- Weight loss. Contrary to popular belief that the banana is fattening, it actually provides one of the most complete meals in history for only 120 calories for a large banana. In my experience it does not do a lot for guilt except you do feel more virtuous eating a banana than a chocolate bar, but it does help with the everyday stress of trying to keep to a healthy eating programme. As weight can be related to stressful environments, a banana also is very good as a work place snack to help you get through the day without resorting to more unhealthy comfort foods.
- Morning sickness and hangovers are hopefully not connected but both these afflictions take place in the morning when blood sugar levels are likely to be low. Eating a banana is said to help stabilise this and if you blend your banana with some milk and honey you will also soothe and hydrate your body whilst calming the stomach.
- Smoking cigarettes is one of those habits that really needs to be given up. It is hard though and I know having gone through the withdrawal symptoms myself 21 years ago. If you can manage without a nicotine patch, you might think about including a banana in your diet everyday or when you have a craving. Not only will all the nutrients give you an energy boost but also the potassium and magnesium in the banana will help with your withdrawal symptoms including stress.
- For warts and mosquito bites there are some old fashioned remedies that are worth mentioning. It is said that if you wrap the inside of the banana skin around a wart that it will disappear and it is reported that rubbing the inside of the skin over mosquito bites will take down the swelling and irritation.

As you can see the banana is a very useful ally in efforts to prevent illness and to help our bodies fight conditions when they occur. It is not the complete answer, as it needs to be included in a diet that contains all the essential elements. It is also not intended to take the place of necessary medication for serious illnesses. It is part of the wonderful pharmacy that we have available at our fingertips and should be enjoyed in as many ways as possible.

Cranberry

Most of us before the 80's restricted cranberries in our diet to Christmas and the odd time we had turkey at other times in the year. Then came the very welcome news that for those of us, who suffered from attacks of bacterial cystitis, drinking the juice of these tart little red berries could bring relief.

In fact emerging evidence shows that this fruit is a lot more versatile than we thought and there are now several very good reasons to include cranberries on a daily basis in your diet. Other berries are now emerging commercially that claim to have more antioxidants than cranberries and certainly it is worth considering including them in your diet on a regular basis. Personally I use cranberry juice on a daily basis and have found that combined with all the other fresh foods that I eat, I have enjoyed an excellent protection from infections such as colds and flu.

Cranberries were used by the Native American Indians as a nutritious addition to their diet and they normally sweetened the cooked berries with honey. Colonists, who had been introduced to the berry, exported it home to England at the beginning of the 18th century. The Indians also used the berries in poultices for wounds as they recognised the antibacterial and antibiotic effect of the fruit even if they could not scientifically prove these properties.

Artery Health

Cranberries are an excellent source of antioxidants which, if you remember from the nutrients section, keep our system clear of damaging free radicals. In the same way, flavanoids in Cranberries function as very potent antioxidants and may reduce the risk of atherosclerosis.

Atherosclerosis is when the arteries become clogged and narrowed restricting blood flow to the heart. The most common cause is a build up of LDL (Low-Density lipoproteins or lousy cholesterol) oxidising and causing plaque to cling to the walls of the arteries narrowing and hardening them. This can lead to angina, blood clots and heart attacks.

Cranberries contain the flavanoids and also polyphenolic compounds that have been shown to help prevent the LDL from oxidising and therefore forming the dangerous plaque that leads to arterial disease.

Dental Health – Another Good Reason to Drink Cranberry Juice

When I left secretarial college, intent on a career on the stage, I took a job as a dental receptionist, which evolved, into my training as a dental nurse.

Canned drinks were becoming all the rage in the 60's and I saw first hand the corrosive damage that these sugary concoctions could inflict on tooth enamel. There was not the kind of education, products or electric toothbrushes in those days, but if there had been more of one type of drink around in those days we would have seen a lot less decay.

One would think that drinking cranberry juice with its natural sugars would have a harmful effect on the teeth but in fact the reverse is true. Cranberries actually help prevent dental problems.

A study published in the Journal of the American Dental Association reported that there is a unique component in cranberry juice, which is technically termed High molecular weight non-dialysable material or NDM for short. Hundreds of different types of bacteria in the mouth clump together and attach themselves to the teeth and gums and over time hardens causing cavities and gum disease. This film on the teeth becomes resistant to saliva, which would normally remove bacteria from the mouth and also our normal oral hygiene routines such as brushing. One of the most resistant bacteria in the mouth is Streptococcus and in tests indications showed that Cranberry mouthwash reduced the presence of this in the mouth significantly.

NDM in cranberries has the power to prevent this bacteria build-up in the first place having a long-term effect on your dental health.

Other fruits were tested including Blueberries which as we have discussed is part of the same family as cranberries but the NDM was in much weaker concentrations in these and all other fruits tested.

So whilst you need to visit your dentist regularly, in between visits to have your teeth cleaned, drink cranberry juice and prevent the build up of plaque and avoid further damage to your teeth.

Cranberry Juice And Peptic Ulcers

A peptic ulcer is a sore on the lining of the stomach or duodenum, which is the beginning of the small intestine. They are quite common and one of the main causes is bacterial infection and the chief culprit is Helicobacter Pylori (H.Pylori). It is not certain how people contract H.Pylori but it is believed that 20% of people under 40 and half of the population over 60 are infected with it.

H. Pylori weakens the protective mucous coating of the stomach and duodenum, which allows acid to get through to the sensitive lining beneath. Both the acid and the bacteria irritate the lining causing a sore or ulcer. H. Pylori are able to survive in stomach acid because it secretes enzymes that neutralise the acid. Once in the safety of the mucous lining the bacteria's spiral shape allows it to burrow into the lining.

H. Pylori have also been associated with stomach cancer, acid reflux and gastritis. Finding a natural way to prevent H. pylori from completing its mission is therefore a very prime research topic.

As in dental health the NDM (high molecular weight non-dialysable) prevents the H.Pylori from attaching itself to the lining of the stomach therefore preventing an ulcer developing.

Other Benefits of Cranberries

Emerging research is indicating that the benefits of cranberries is even more far reaching with research into its anti-viral properties in the treatment of genital herpes, prevention of kidney infections and kidney stones. What is extremely interesting is the cranberries ability to inhibit the growth of common food related pathogens including Listeria and E.Coli 0157:H7. This antibiotic effect of cranberries was recognised centuries ago by the American Indians and it is a pity that we are only just catching up with these enlightened people.

How to Eat Cranberries

By far the best way to get your daily fix of cranberries is fresh, mixed with other fruit or juiced. They are very tart however and

I compromise by drinking the light version of the cranberry juice when the fruit is out of season.

The recommended ration of cranberry juice is two 10 oz glasses per day. One in the morning and one in the evening it takes two hours for the antibacterial properties to be effective and they then last approximately twelve hours.

Oranges

Apart from the obvious of being juicy and sweet, oranges have a number of healthy benefits – primarily their high Vitamin C concentration. Just one orange supplies over 100% of your daily requirement of vitamin C.

The orange's high level of fibre also helps with the cholesterol. It obviously helps with digestion but can also affect and lower blood sugar levels. This means that even diabetics can eat them. The fibre in oranges has also been shown to stabilise intestinal problems such as constipation and diarrhoea and is great for people suffering from chronic problems such as IBS.

Along with apple juice and grapefruit juice – drinking orange juice can help prevent kidney stones from forming as it increases urinary pH value and citric acid excretion which is necessary to prevent the forming of calcium deposits that become kidney stones.

Other areas that oranges have been shown to benefit us are with ulcers.

Apart from vitamin C, oranges also contain folic acid, potassium as well as calcium and magnesium.

Vegetables

Asparagus

We are all aware today of the health benefits of eating fresh fruit and vegetables but for thousands of years humans have not only taken nourishment from natural foods but have also utilised many parts of the plant for medicinal purposes.

We have an abundance of fresh produce in Spain all year round and this includes asparagus.

What Is the History of Asparagus?

Asparagus is a member of the lily family and the spears that we eat are shoots grown underground. The Greeks cultivated the plant in the eastern Mediterranean area over 2,500 years ago using it fresh in season and dried during the winter months. The Romans regarded asparagus a great delicacy and there is evidence that they would transport the new season's crop to the Alps where it was frozen and stored until required.

It has always been prized for its medicinal properties and was used for urinary tract and kidney problems as well as a natural diuretic. Anyone who has consumed a plate of freshly cooked asparagus will have noticed that the after affects include very pungent urine.

What Gives Asparagus its Health Benefits?

Everyone knows that eating a diet rich in antioxidants will boost you immune system but asparagus has a few other nutrients that are special. One of these is inulin which feeds our friendly bacteria in the intestine and prevents the harmful variety from taking over.

It contains Vitamin K which is the subject of a great deal of research into not just blood clotting but also as a preventative for heart disease and osteoporosis and it may turn out to be one of the strongest antioxidants in the fight against cancer.

Japan has even approved Vitamin K for the treatment of osteoporosis and along with the calcium and phosphorus in Asparagus makes this vegetable an essential in any middle-aged person's diet.

If you don't want to lose your marbles as you get older then eating a regular serving of asparagus will help prevent inflammation in the brain which leads to dementia. This anti-inflammatory effect also eases the inflammation of the joints.

A deficiency of vitamin K has been linked to elevated levels of blood sugar, as the pancreas, which makes insulin normally, contains the second highest amount of vitamin K than anywhere in the body.

What Other Nutrients Does Asparagus Offer Us?

As well as Vitamin K, asparagus also contains high levels of Folate a B vitamin that is very important for the reproductive system. It helps prevent birth defects so eating asparagus frequently during the week should be part of your eating plan prior to becoming pregnant. In addition Folate is great for heart health.

On an every day basis the other nutrients including Vitamin C, A, B1, B2, B3, B6, Tryptophan, Manganese, Copper, Phosphorus, potassium, iron, zinc, magnesium, selenium, and calcium make this a very powerful healing food. Great for water retention, healthy intestinal flora and immune system.

As with all fresh fruit and vegetables the antioxidants in asparagus such as Vitamin A, C and selenium have an overall benefit for the body. I cannot keep stressing the importance of a healthy immune system enough. One area that is going to increase in concern is MRSA. This is the resistant strain of bacteria that is causing such upheaval in health care facilities. Sick people in hospitals have weak immune systems and it leaves them very vulnerable to these infections. My philosophy is that if you have a very healthy immune system you rarely become sick anyway. Accidents however are unavoidable especially with the elderly who might fall and require replacement hip or other joint surgery. If the elderly person eats well and has a healthy immune system when they undergo the surgery they are far less likely to contract MRSA. If you have elective surgery planned and you have several weeks or months to wait on the list, use it to your advantage. Build your immune system up before you go in and you will improve your recovery rate as well as help protect yourself from disease.

What Is the Best Way to Prepare Asparagus?

Cut off the fibrous base before cooking, as this can be tough and difficult to digest. Make sure it is thoroughly washed. Tie the stalks together with cooking twine and either boil the whole bundle or stand it upright in boiling water in a special asparagus pan so that the tender tips steam and the tougher stalks boil. I also use one of the electronic steamers and this leaves the shoots tender and colourful.

You can roast with other vegetables such as red peppers, onions and mushrooms in a little olive oil.

Sauté chopped asparagus with shitake mushrooms and turkey and add to a little brown rice.

Serve hot or cold with a spinach and walnut salad.

Aubergine

We were all encouraged to eat our 'greens' when we were children, and although I cannot recollect being told to eat my 'purples' it is this colour which gives this healing food its uniqueness.

When we enjoy a moussaka or ratatouille made with this versatile food we don't tend to dwell on its medicinal properties, but like the majority of fresh produce we eat aubergines have some powerful health benefits.

The aubergine has its origins in India, and in ancient Sanskrit was called 'Vatinganah'. The Persians changed this to 'Badingan' and around 1,500 years ago it is thought that the Moors brought the 'al-badhinjan' to Spain with them. The Spaniards thought that the article 'al' was part of the word, so it went into the language as alberginia. The French finally picked this up as aubergine.

The English name, eggplant, arose in the eighteenth century to describe the white, or yellowish, goose-egg-size fruits that were more common than the now-familiar deep purple colour.

In Spain, today, aubergines are called berengenas or 'apples of love' for their supposed aphrodisiac properties. In northern Europe they had a strange notion that eating aubergines caused fevers and epileptic seizures and named it Mala Insana or 'mad apple'.

The aubergine belongs to the nightshade family that includes tomatoes, sweet peppers and potatoes. It grows from a vine and the fruits vary in size and colour. Its flesh tends to be slightly bitter and spongy in texture.

When you are selecting aubergines go for the smaller, smooth skinned fruits. Gently push with your thumb and if the flesh gives slightly, but springs back, it is ripe. If the indentation remains it is overripe and will be soggy inside. If you knock on the fruit and it sounds hollow it will be too dry and inedible.

What Are the Medicinal Properties of the Aubergine?

As with all plants, the aubergine has a sophisticated defence system to ensure its survival. When we eat it, we inherit some of these properties and our bodies' process and use specific nutrients to benefit our own health. The aubergine has an abundance of nutrients and antioxidants. Two especially important nutrients are, Nasunin, a flavanoid, and the phenolic compound chlorogenic acid.

Nasunin is a potent antioxidant in the skin of the aubergine and has been studied for its ability to prevent free radical damage to cell membranes. Lipids, or fats, are the main component of cell membranes and not only protect the cell from damage but also regulate the passage of nutrients and waste in and out of the cell. Nasunin may also help prevent oxidative damage to the LDL (bad cholesterol) in our blood that can lead to plaque and blockages in the arteries.

Nasunin also assists with the regulation of iron in the body. Iron is essential for both the transportation of oxygen in the blood and for our immune function. However, too much iron can increase free radical damage and is linked to heart disease, cancer and degenerative joint diseases such as rheumatoid arthritis. Nasunin is an iron 'chelator', which means that it binds with iron and transports it safely through the bloodstream preventing any excess from causing damage to cells.

Chlorogenic acid is a phenolic compound and one of the most potent free radical scavengers in plant tissues. It is very abundant in aubergines and very effective in preventing free radical damage to cholesterol. Additionally, it may help prevent certain cancers and viral infections. Like Brussels sprouts, some varieties of aubergine can be very bitter and it is thought that this is due to very high levels of Chlorogenic acid, which is also responsible for the rapid browning of the flesh when it has been cut.

More Good Reasons to Include Aubergine in Your Diet

The aubergine is a good source of dietary fibre. This helps prevent constipation, speeds the elimination of waste from the body and can block the build up of plaque in the bloodstream – which could lead to arterial disease. Recent research is identifying some very interesting properties in certain fibres, including the ability to absorb and eliminate harmful bacteria from the body without the need for antibiotics. Fibre in the diet has also been shown to reduce the risk of colon cancer and to regulate blood sugar levels.

By eating aubergines regularly you will also be absorbing; Potassium, Manganese, Copper, Vitamins B1, B3, B6, Folate, Magnesium and Tryptophan.

Some current research on brain cell health suggests that eating aubergines regularly may help protect us from degenerative brain diseases such as Alzheimer's.

Are There Any Drawbacks to Eating Aubergines?

The majority of us can enjoy aubergines on a regular basis and obtain its full health benefits, but a small proportion of people should avoid eating it.

The aubergine contains relatively high concentrations of oxalates, which are found in all plants and humans. If oxalates are too concentrated they can crystallise and form stones in the kidneys and the gallbladder. If you suffer from kidney or gallbladder problems then it would be best to avoid aubergines. This caution also applies to anyone who suffers from rheumatoid arthritis or gout, as this vegetable is part of the nightshade family and could increase the symptoms of these diseases.

It is important to remember that variety is the spice of life. Including many different foods in your diet ensures that you get a broad spectrum of nutrients and health benefits from as many different sources as possible.

Brussel Sprouts

Our immune system is very efficient but life takes its toll. It is important that in our diet we include foods that enhance and boost our immune system and the Brussel sprout does just that.

Brussel sprouts contain a phytochemical, which helps our own defence system to protect against disease in general but in particular cancer. Sulforaphane is a phytonutrient found in this group of plant families helps boost the body's detoxification enzymes, which help clear carcinogenic substances from the body quickly and efficiently. Brussel sprouts have also been shown to decrease the level of DNA damage in cells, which prevents mutations in the cells, which allows cancer to develop.

To get the benefit of this phytochemical the food needs to be chopped or chewed so that the liver is stimulated into producing the specific detoxification enzymes and research has shown that breast cancer cells particularly are preventing from reproducing even in later stages of the disease.

Apart from cancer the Brussel sprout and other members of the Brassica family such as cabbage, cauliflower and broccoli contain large amounts of vitamin C. This supports our immune function and has been shown to help prevent heart disease, strokes and cancer but also promotes the manufacture of collagen, a protein that forms the body structure including the skin, connective tissues and cartilage. A serving of Brussel sprouts also contains very healthy quantities of Vitamin A and beta-carotene, both vital in defending the body and promoting healthy and young looking skin.

Birth Defects

Folic acid has long been recognised for its ability to help protect the foetus against birth defects. Folic acid is a B vitamin that promotes healthy cell division. Without it nervous system cells do not divide properly which has linked to a number of birth defects such as spina bifida. The main source of folic acid is green leafy vegetables such as the Brussel sprout and spinach but as our reliance on processed foods rather than fresh fruit and vegetables grows, the deficiency of this vitamin is becoming the most common in the western world.

Other Benefits

Apart from being rich in fibre, which helps protect us against colon disease this vegetable because of its high content of antioxidants, particularly vitamin C, is a great preventative for degenerative diseases such as rheumatoid arthritis.

How to Prepare

Wash, trim and remove the outer leaves of the sprouts. To preserve all the nutrients use a steamer to cook the sprouts until tender.

Season and drizzle with a little olive oil and add an extra nutritional boost by adding some chopped almonds or walnuts before you serve.

Cabbage

This versatile vegetable has a very distinguished medical history dating back over 4000 years and was considered by the ancient Greeks and other European natural healers to be the ultimate medicine. It has been used internally and externally in the treatment of gangrene, rheumatism, respiratory conditions, gastritis, bladder inflammation, peptic ulcers, ulcerative colitis, IBS and cancer. The list is virtually endless and there are many recipes in folklore for the preparation of the vegetable.

Apparently the most potent way to take your cabbage daily is in the form of juice but having tasted some it does benefit by the addition of a couple of other nutritious ingredients, namely carrots and apples. Honey is also used adding its healing properties for respiratory problems.

What Are the Nutrients in Cabbage?

From a nutritional perspective, cabbage is very high in Vitamin C but also has good amounts of fibre, B vitamins, Omega 3 fatty acids, some calcium, potassium and magnesium. It is of course a low calorie food and you can eat a generous serving gaining all the nutrients but only 30 calories.

Much of current research is centred on the phytochemicals in cabbage in relation to cancer research and there is evidence that suggests eating cabbage and other members of the Brassica family such as broccoli, cauliflower and Brussel sprouts could lower your risk of getting cancer. It would appear that the phytochemicals help activate the antioxidant and detoxification processes that remove and destroy cancer-producing substances.

For example there was a very interesting study conducted over a period of years which could lead to some breakthroughs in the prevention of breast cancer.

Cabbage may be at the heart of why the breast cancer risk of Polish women triples after they immigrate to the United States, rising to match the rate of U.S.-born women. A few years ago a Dr. Pathak from the University of New Mexico revealed the results of a study that she and her team had been conducting.

Young women, who eat four or more servings per week of raw or lightly cooked cabbage, such as coleslaw or steamed sauerkraut, may significantly reduce their risk of breast cancer later in life. This is the way that cabbage is traditionally served in Poland.

Compared with women who ate 1.5 servings or less of cabbage per week during adolescence, those who ate four or more servings were 72% less likely to develop breast cancer as adults. We already know that cabbage contains anti-carcinogenic glucosinolates and myrosinase enzymes but this research is one of the most conclusive studies and hopefully it will expanded to provide some concrete evidence of the power of this very simple and readily available vegetable.

Women who consumed low amounts of cabbage in their teens could still derive some protective benefit from cabbage if they increased their consumption during adulthood so including cabbage three or four times a week is an excellent idea.

How About Preparing Cabbage in the Healthiest Way?

There are a number of ways to incorporate cabbage into your everyday healthy eating plan and one of the best ways of course is to eat it raw. Make sure that the cabbage is firm with brightly coloured leaves and the darker green the better. Wash carefully to remove any contaminants and unwanted guests. Soaking in salty water for 15 minutes and then rinsing usually gets rid of insects. Do not buy cut vegetables of any kind as they lose many of their nutrients, particularly vitamin C as soon as they are cut.

You can shred cabbage and add to the other Brassica family vegetables, broccoli florets and cauliflower and make a raw vegetable salad. Mixed with carrot and onion and a spoonful of mayonnaise, coleslaw is an accompaniment not only for salads but also for fish and lean meats. It is said that a salad of cabbage and apple with some lemon juice cures a hangover but this is one I have not tried. It is delicious in stir-fry and you can use the Chinese cabbage in this recipe

If you cook cabbage you will be removing many of its nutrients so steaming is the best option. To make a cabbage juice you will need either an electric juicer or you can liquidise and then strain through a sieve.

Cabbage and potato soup is delicious as are the variations using carrot and other root vegetables. Bubble and squeak is a favourite dish for children and will encourage them to include this unprepossessing but powerful vegetable in their diet.

Carrots

(Now you will see why the carrot is part of the title of this book!)

The humble carrot is a vegetable most of us take for granted. Like many of the foods included here, carrots have an ancient history, originating in of all places Afghanistan. The Greeks and the Romans ate carrots and in fact the Greeks called the carrot 'Philtron' and used it as an aphrodisiac. Perhaps we won't go into that in too much detail but apparently it made men more ardent and women more yielding.

In Asia the carrot was an established root crop and was then introduced to Europe in the 13th century. It was the Middle Ages before the carrot became better known and doctors of the time prescribed carrots for numerous ills including snakebite. In those days the carrot was available in far more radiant colours including red, purple, black, yellow and white. They were cultivated together and over time it resulted in the orange vegetable we know today.

The Elizabethans on receiving the carrots from mainland Europe did some rather strange things with them. Some ate the roots but others used the feathery foliage for decoration in hats and on their clothes. I am sure like every fashion statement this may come and revisit us at some point. The colonists took the carrot to America but they were not really cultivated there until the last couple of centuries.

What Are the Health Benefits of Carrots?

Carrots eaten as fresh, raw and unprocessed food are full of nutrients including Vitamin A, beta carotene (turned into Vitamin A in the body), other carotenoids, B Vitamins, Vitamin C and minerals calcium and potassium. Of all of the nutrients Beta-Carotene and latterly Alpha Carotene are seen as the most important properties of the carrot.

Beta-carotene is one of about 500 compounds called carotenoids, which are present in most fruit and vegetables. The body changes beta-carotene into Vitamin A, which promotes a healthy immune system and healthy cell growth. The body can only change so much beta-carotene into Vitamin A and any excess also boosts the immune system and is a powerful antioxidant in its own right. Antioxidants prevent free radical damage to cells, tissues and most importantly to the fat in our bloodstream that can lead to blocked arteries and heart disease.

Alpha carotene has often been overlooked in carrots but some interesting studies in Japan indicate that Alpha carotene might be even more powerful than Beta-carotene in the fight against cancer.

Acidity in the Body

Carrots play an important role in neutralising acid in the body. Many common conditions that we suffer from are due to excess acid in the body including indigestion, peptic ulcers, urinary tract infections, arthritis, and cancer.

Too much acid will decrease the energy production in the cells and the ability to repair damaged cells. The body is unable to detox heavy metals and that allows tumour cells to thrive. It will also cause a depressed immune system leaving the body wide open to infections.

Being mildly acidic can cause headaches, stomach problems and general fatigue but if the body continues to accumulate acid in tissues and bloodstream far more serious health problems will develop such as degenerative diseases and cancer.

Carrot is an alkaline forming food that works with the pH in your body to ensure that safe levels are maintained.

Apart from neutralising the overall acidity in your body, one of the areas that eating carrots or drinking carrot juice may help you is with acid stomach and it would certainly be healthier for you than consuming packets of antacid tablets. If you are suffering from urinary tract infections where the urine is acidic, carrot juice combined with cranberry juice (to prevent the adhesion of bacteria to the soft tissues) will help speed your recovery.

What Is the Best Way to Prepare Carrots?

As with any fresh food it is much better for you to eat carrots raw so that you lose none of the nutrients during cooking. If you are going to eat them cooked then steam them or roast them with vegetables such as courgettes, aubergines and onions with olive oil and herbs.,

On a final note, we often feed carrots to horses as a treat but in fact racehorse breeders use carrots as part of the normal diet to increase performance and health in their animals. Who knows, if you start including more carrots in your diet you may be eligible for the Grand National next year.

Mushrooms

This common food is not only nutritious but has also been used as a healing food for 1000's of years, particularly in the East. Supermarkets all over the world are now supplying more and more exotic varieties and they should be included in your weekly shopping.

In the past it has been usual to eliminate mushrooms from the diet if you have a fungal infection such as Candida. True, mushrooms are a fungus, but they are too powerful a source of nutrients and healing properties to exclude completely on a permanent basis. Studies even suggest that they are probiotic encouraging the body to produce healthy bacteria in the intestines, which is exactly what is needed in the treatment of Candida.

More and more research is indicating that certain varieties have the overwhelming potential to cure cancer and AIDS and in Japan some of the extracts from mushrooms are already being used in mainstream medicine.

There are an estimated 20,000 varieties of mushrooms with around 2,000 being edible. Of these over 250 types of mushroom have been recognised as being medically active or therapeutic.

Apart from their medicinal properties, mushrooms are first and foremost an excellent food source. They are low in calories, high in B vitamins, Vitamin C, calcium, iron phosphorus, potassium, zinc and supply us with protein and fibre. They are versatile and they are easy to cook and blend with other ingredients on a daily basis. For vegetarians they provide not only protein but also the daily recommended amount of B12 a vitamin often lacking in a non-meat diet.

Although we associate modern medicinal mushrooms with Japan they in fact were used extensively in both diet and healing in Ancient Egypt and Rome where they were regarded as gifts from the gods. 3,000 years ago certain varieties of mushrooms were used in Chinese medicine and they still play a huge role in Chinese cuisine today.

The Link to Antibiotics

Although I am anti the over use of antibiotics, there is no doubt that their discovery by Sir Alexander Fleming saved countless lives in wartime and since.

This fantastic breakthrough and the development of most of our modern antibiotics such as tetracycline, auremycin and cyclosporin were all derived from fungus. Without some of these drugs not only would millions die from bacterial infections but we would be unable to transplant hearts or other organs. For example, Cyclosporin is used to suppress the immune system in transplant patients to prevent rejection.

Mushrooms in General

The most common mushrooms that you are likely to use in cookery are white button mushrooms and oyster mushrooms. They may not be as exotic as some of the oriental varieties but they still hold many health benefits. Not only are they low in calories and fat which is great if you are trying to lose weight but also will provide you with plenty of fibre. Even the little white mushrooms contain B vitamins, potassium and selenium and there are some interesting studies being conducted at the moment into some very important health benefits.

One area of research is into the phytochemical action that suppresses two enzymes, aromatase and steroid 5alpha-reductase. Aromatase converts the hormone androgen into oestrogen, an excess of which can promote the development of breast cancer. Steroid 5alpha-reductase has the same effect on testosterone converting it to dihydrotestosterone, which has been shown to be involved in the development of prostate cancer. In the laboratory the team led by a Dr. Chen discovered that the mushroom extract suppressed the growth of both these cells.

Another property in mushrooms that is potentially very interesting is the amount of the antioxidant ergothioneine compared to the amounts in other foods such as wheat germ and chicken livers. In fact mushrooms can have up to 12 times as much which means that a small serving of 5 oz could provide excellent protection against oxidative damage throughout the body.

There are two medicinal mushrooms that you will find either fresh in your supermarket or dried in your health food shop. Shiitake and Maitake mushrooms have been used for thousands of years and they are definitely worth including in your diet several times per week.

Shiitake Mushrooms

Shiitake mushrooms range in colour from tan to dark brown with broad umbrella shaped caps. They are soft and spongy in texture and when cooked are rich tasting and meaty in texture. They are ideal as an alternative to red meat in pasta dishes as you can chop them finely and cook with a little olive oil in exactly the same way.

Shiitake's main benefit is the ability to lower cholesterol. There is a specific amino acid in the mushroom, which helps speed up the processing of cholesterol in the liver resulting in lower levels in the blood.

In 1969 Japanese scientists isolated a polysaccharide (sugar) compound from Shiitake they called Lentinan. It appears that this substance stimulates the immune system cells to rid the body of tumour cells resulting in either a reduction in size or complete removal of cancerous growths. In Japan the Federal Drug Agency has licensed Lentinan as an anti-cancer drug and it would be great if the American and European agencies would catch up with this different approach in the East.

AIDS sufferers have to take a complex cocktail of drugs to minimise the development of the disease but in trials an extract from the Shiitake (LEM or Lentinula edodes myucelium) was more effective then AZT. In test tubes this extract blocked the HIV cells from reproducing and damaging immune system cells. It was also effective against some of the more common viral infections that AIDS patients develop such as Herpes.

The liver is very robust but certain viruses, especially Hepatitis B, can affect it very badly. LEM has been tested and it was found that in a limited trial that it stimulated the body to produce antibodies to the virus. Hopefully this research will continue and more definitive evidence produced.

Maitake

The Maitake mushroom is found in clusters of dark fronds, which are firm but supple at the base. They have a distinctive aroma and taste rich and earthy. They are great in any dish where you use mushrooms but are wonderful in a homemade stroganoff sauce served with brown rice.

They are also known as the "hen of the woods" possibly because of their shape. As with the Shiitake this mushroom has a compound that inhibits the growth of cancer cells by stimulating the immune system and in addition they have been found to lower blood pressure and blood cholesterol levels but this has not been proven in humans as yet.

Another area of research is diabetes and it is thought that Maitake mushrooms may have a blood sugar balancing action that may reduce the need for insulin.

As you can see mushrooms as with most fruit and vegetables hold some interesting and potentially life saving properties. The pity is that the Ancients knew of these properties and put them to good use. Now we have to invent the wheel all over again and hope that someone will finance the research to prove not only that they work but that it is worth developing them into lifesaving drugs.

Onion and Garlic

The onion is part of the Lily family which includes garlic, leeks, welsh onions and chives. The word onion comes from the old English word unyun derived from the French word oignon which in turn came from the Latin unio. There are words for the vegetable in ancient languages but none seem to be related to each other indicating how widespread the use of it was.

Onions have been used for thousands of years as a seasoning for otherwise bland food and today we can buy them all year round and use them raw or cooked in a wide variety of dishes.

What Are the Health Benefits of Onions?

The onion contains a powerful sulphur containing compound which is responsible for the pungent odour and for the health benefits. Onions contain allyl propyl disulphide, chromium, Vitamin C and flavanoids, the most beneficial being quercitin.

Allyl propyl disulphide lowers blood sugar levels by competing with insulin which is also a disulphide for space in the liver where insulin is normally deactivated. This results in an increase in the amount of insulin available to move glucose into cells causing a lowering of blood sugar.

Chromium helps cells respond efficiently to insulin which in turn decreases blood sugar levels. These two properties in the onion make it a vegetable worth including in our daily diet as we get older to help prevent the onset of Type 2 diabetes.

Chromium has also been shown to improve glucose tolerance,

lower insulin levels, decrease total cholesterol levels whilst increasing levels of the healthy cholesterol (HDL).

The reduction in cholesterol levels leads to reductions in blood pressure levels which is of course a leading cause of cardiovascular disease. Eating onions with other foods with high levels of bioflavanoids (tea, apples, broccoli, cranberry juice etc) has been proven to reduce the risk of heart disease

Quercitin combined with Vitamin C work together to kill bacteria which is why they are so valuable added to soups and stews during the cold and flu season.

There are other areas where eating onions regularly can reduce your risk on developing degenerative and sometimes life threatening diseases. These include Colon cancer, osteo and rheumatoid arthritis, asthma and other inflammatory diseases.

An exciting area of research into bone health had identified that a compound in onions with a mile long name but GPCS for short may inhibit the activity of osteoclasts which are the cells that break down bone. The implication is that for women this may be a safe and natural alternative to some of the prescribed medication given to women during the menopause to prevent osteoporosis. This obviously does not mean that you should cease taking your medication but you could begin including onions in your diet several times a week and if your doctor is satisfied that your bone density levels can be maintained, you may be able to reduce or cease using the medication.

Onions also contain healthy amounts of other nutrients such as manganese, Vitamin B6, tryptophan, folate, potassium, phosphorus and copper making onions a superfood.

Garlic

The garlic is a multi-bulb cousin to the onion. Again originating in Asia it has been used for thousands of years as a pungent additive to food but also as a healing agent. In recent years its reputation has been validated by hundreds of research studies and like the onion it is worth including in your diet very regularly.

Garlic contains many helpful compounds including thiosulfinates such as allicin, sulphates including alliin and dithins the most researched being ajoene.

Research has identified that garlic lowers blood pressure; decreases the ability of platelets to clump together forming clots, reduces blood levels of lousy cholesterol (LDL) whilst increasing levels of healthy cholesterol (HDL). It also helps our blood vessels relax which prevents atherosclerosis, heart disease and the risks of heart attacks and strokes.

Garlic, like the onion is anti-inflammatory, anti-bacterial and anti-viral and what is interesting garlic appears to be an effective antibiotic, even against some of the resistant strains such as MRSA.

Cancer protection is essential for all of us. The compound ajoene seems to be effective in the treatment of skin cancer and eating two or more servings a week of garlic may help prevent colon cancer.

Allicin has also been researched in regard to weight loss as there are some indications that in the laboratory at least, this compound may inhibit weight gain.

Certainly garlic is a powerful anti-oxidant and as we prepare ourselves for the winter months and the inevitable cold season, taking garlic in our food is not only a tasty way to take a preventative medicine but also an effective one.

I have put together some recipes for onions and garlic that are easy to prepare and that you can include in your diet two or three times a week to maximise the effect of these two great superfoods and you will find these later in the book.

Spinach

Spinach actually has more nutrients than any other food if you compare it calorie for calorie. It has excellent amounts of all the B vitamins, Vitamin K, manganese, folate, iron, potassium and magnesium.

Spinach has the highest level of chlorophyll the substances that stimulate haemoglobin and red blood cell production. Since this process is vital to ensure adequate supplies of oxygen are delivered to all parts of the body it works hand in hand with lung function.

Diseases that spinach and other dark green leafy vegetables helps protect us against read like a medical dictionary but there is growing evidence that it works particularly well against various types of cancer including of the lungs.

The History of Spinach

Spinach originates in Asia, probably Iran where it was known as "aspanakh" and it came to Europe in the 1300's. It was primarily used in religious ceremonies, particularly during Lent but by the

1800's it was being cultivated and bears the distinction of being our first frozen vegetable.

What Other Health Benefits Does Spinach Offer?

Spinach contains many different flavanoids, which are highly effective antioxidants and anti-cancer agents. Research is ongoing into the use of concentrated spinach extracts that could be used in conjunction with more conventional treatments with the benefit of the usual side effects. The possible action of these flavanoids is to slow down the division of cancer cells in a number of areas of the body including the breast and prostate.

We have already covered the essential health benefits of including Vitamin K in our diet and eating spinach provides us with an abundant source containing one of the highest levels of this vitamin providing over 1000% of our daily requirement.

Our hearts are very vulnerable to oxidative damage and the high levels of Vitamin A and Vitamin C in spinach offer fantastic protection. Additionally the folate levels in spinach are excellent so this will mean a reduction in homocysteine in the blood. Homocysteine is a very harmful chemical and a great deal of evidence points to this as being one of the main causes of heart disease and strokes.

Properties of spinach that are age specific are the Vitamin C for repair and maintenance of the blood vessels, lutein to protect against age-related eye degeneration and iron for energy.

Eating spinach will help reduce stress, boost your immune system, help lower your blood pressure, reduce your risk of developing cancer, and is also an anti-inflammatory agent for arthritis and asthma.

How to Use Spinach

Spinach is wonderful raw and you will not lose any of these fantastic nutrients. Wash thoroughly and then put in salads or use as a garnish for main courses. Add to sandwiches instead of lettuce.

Sauté with olive oil, onions and garlic and use as a dressing for jacket potatoes. Put into soups, omelettes and pasta dishes.

A Word of Warning

Whilst the majority of people can enjoy Spinach several times per week there are a few individuals with specific problems who should avoid it. Still include other dark green leafy vegetables on a regular basis but monitor your main symptoms and check for reactions within 12 to 24 hours after eating them.

Oxalates are a naturally occurring substance in plants, animals and humans. If there is too high a concentration in the bloodstream it can crystallise and cause problems for people who suffer from kidney or gallbladder problems. It also contains purines, which are broken down to form uric acid, the cause of gout and kidney stones.

Watercress

The Latin name of watercress is Nasturtium officinale and it is part of the mustard family

Watercress history goes back over three thousand years to the Persians, Greeks and Romans. In the past it has been used as a breath freshener and palate cleanser as well as for its medicinal properties. Apparently Captain Cook included it in his sailors' diet to combat scurvy and there are rumours that it is an aphrodisiac. But, before you all rush out to get your packet of watercress we better cover some of this lovely green vegetable's other health benefits.

What Is the Nutritional Content of Watercress?

Like all fresh fruit and vegetables Watercress has generous amounts of Vitamins A, C and E, which of course are fantastic antioxidants and it also contains calcium, folic acid and iron, all nutrients that I have covered earlier. Some interesting facts are that watercress contains more iron than spinach, more calcium than milk, has three times as much vitamin E as lettuce and has 150% more folic acid than broccoli.

What Are its Health Benefits of Watercress?

Well, apart from obviously providing a great nutritional fix every time you eat it, there are certain illnesses that watercress has been used for during the centuries. Some of the more common ones are cataracts, coronary heart disease, lung and breast cancers and hormone related cancers.

Eating it regularly along with the other dark green leafy vegetables in the healthy eating plan may help reduce your LDL cholesterol levels, help PMS or menopausal problems, lower blood pressure and also boost your immune system.

Some other older cultures have used watercress extensively since there was no pharmacy around the corner and they make interesting reading.

- The Romans treated insanity with vinegar and watercress (you may have stayed mad but your lips were so puckered you stopped raving) Apparently Roman emperors ate watercress to help them make 'bold decisions'.
- Eating a bag of watercress is meant to cure a hangover.
- Brazilian researchers found that the extract of watercress appeared to possess anti-tumour properties and it was active against TB.
- Irish monks were said to survive on watercress sandwiches, which may have been because on holy islands there was no supermarket, let alone a pharmacy!
- In the 17th century it was used to cleanse the blood (much more pleasant that blood letting)

In general, watercress has traditionally been considered as a diuretic, expectorant, purgative and stimulant and considered ideal for anaemia, eczema, migraines, toothache, kidney and liver complaints, TB, skin conditions such as warts and of course tumours.

How to Use Watercress

It is a lovely fresh flavour used raw in salads. Put a handful in with your lettuce and spinach and it adds another colour to your leaf vegetables.

Wash carefully and then eat in a sandwich with wholemeal bread. In the Second World War, watercress sandwiches and vinegar was a staple supper on Sunday nights. A lovely variation on this is boiled egg and watercress sandwiches.

As we move into the winter months you can use watercress in homemade vegetable soups, either as a raw fresh garnish or added in the final minutes of cooking.

Protein

Just as you should not remove carbohydrates completely from your diet, you should also not stop eating protein from either animal or plant sources.

Protein is another food group essential for efficient functioning of the human body and needs to be eaten daily.

It would appear that health is improved when protein is combined with whole grains particularly if the protein is vegetable sourced such as in beans which are a combination of the two food groups. Not sure where the food combiners stand on this issue but you will find that many foods we eat have a combination of protein and carbohydrates in varying proportions.

Originally we would have only eaten protein in the form of meat and it is only as we discovered vegetables and grains that these would have been introduced into the diet.

I can from experience tell you that when I removed animal protein from my diet for three years about seventeen years ago, I began to suffer from several soft tissue injuries such as tendon and ligament damage. When I put fish and lean meat back into my diet these problems improved and this despite my careful inclusion of vegetable proteins in my diet.

Some people find that they are healthy on a non animal protein diet but I have worked with several clients who have suffered poor skin and hair health, lack of energy and frequent infections.

If you are considering becoming a vegetarian then I strongly advise you to do careful study first and also make sure that any teenagers you have who suddenly declare they can no longer eat animals do not just stop eating altogether. Growing bodies require protein and you must ensure adequate amounts of vegetable protein are included to compensate for the loss of dairy, meat or fish.

You will find that the healthy eating plan at the back of the book is a combination diet which includes protein with every meal and snack. The carbohydrates are complex and you will not be eating as much as you may have been used to.

As you get to your optimum weight you will reach a point where weight loss plateaus and in my experience you will find yourself automatically reaching for the food you need at any particular time.

For example, I really find it very difficult to eat carbohydrates at night. Not just because I will not be needing them for strenuous activities at that time of day but because I really do not feel like eating them. I am hungry but for lean protein and vegetables.

However, in the morning when I wake up I look forward to my bowl of porridge or muesli and I really could not face a fry up or even a poached egg on toast.

Lunchtime I seem happy to eat rice or potatoes or even a sandwich so it seems to me that my body has reached a point where I am actually listening to its needs and requirements more than I did before.

At first it may seem strange to be eating in this way which is why you will find in the example menus that I have included some cooked breakfasts or carbohydrates in your evening meal until you have adjusted fully to a new way of eating.

In all cases of protein you want to avoid high concentrations of saturated fats and therefore you must remove fat from meat and poultry so that you obtain the full benefits of the protein without too much of the saturated fat.

Include all kinds of lean meat, fish, eggs, dairy and poultry in your programme and eat as much as will fit into your cupped palm as a portion guide.

Dairy Products

Skimmed milk can take a bit of getting used to but in fact you will still get all the benefits including more calcium by using this instead of whole milk or semi-skimmed. However, if you are not looking to lose weight then using either of the alternatives in a balanced way is not a problem.

Cheese is tasty especially when grilled. However, it is high in saturated fats as is butter and during your healthy eating programme it is a good idea to keep away from cheese laden meals and snacks such as Pizza which of course is usually made with white flour anyway.

As you get fitter and healthier and feel you are at your target weight then you can begin to work the 80/20 rule so that you are following the programme 80% of the time with 20% leeway where you can occasionally indulge in a toasted cheese sandwich or piece of pizza.

The problem is today that we have a much higher standard of living and what used to be an occasional treat such as a bar of chocolate on Saturday or a pizza once a month when we went out is now a daily occurrence and considered part of our normal diet.

Get into the habit of regarding suspect foods as occasional entries in your food diary and I can tell you that after a while you will find many of them too sweet, too salty or too fatty for your taste buds.

Butter is better for you than margarine but a scrape of butter still provides you with all the taste and after a while you may even find yourself enjoying a nutty, fresh baked whole grain slice of toast with a drizzle of olive oil and fresh tomatoes sprinkled with basil!

Low fat yoghurts are extremely useful as they can jazz up not only your fruit salad but also savoury dishes that you used to prepare with full fat milk or cream.

I do use low fat cream cheese because I enjoy it and also find it a useful accompaniment to jacket potatoes or even crisp breads and rice cakes.

Drinking green tea will cut down on some of your dairy intake and you can also use a slice of lemon in other teas.

I do not believe in removing all dairy products from the diet as I consider that it has been used by the body to provide elements of essential nutrition for most of our development.

Salmon

There are a number of health issues apart from heart function that eating salmon benefits including weight loss, bone health, a healthy immune system and brain health. The nutrients in this important source of protein are also helpful in preventing cancer and diabetes.

I will begin with Omega 3, which is abundant in fatty fish such as Salmon. Omega-3 (Linolenic Acid) is the principal Omega-3 fatty acid and is used in the formation of cell walls, improving circulation and oxygen. It is important that your overall cholesterol is kept to a normal level but it is equally important to ensure that the balance between the LDL (lousy cholesterol) and the HDL (healthy cholesterol) is maintained with a lower LDL to HDL ratio. Omega 3 appears to maintain that correct balance. An added bonus in eating salmon muscle is that it contains peptides that may also lower blood pressure.

One trial in New Zealand measured adults with a high cholesterol level over a 4-week period. They consumed 3 gm of salmon oil per day and after the 4 weeks they showed an increase of HDL and a decrease in LDL levels. Lowering both cholesterol and blood pressure levels certainly contributes to a healthy heart.

Omega 3 is linked to brain health in a number of ways. The brain contains a large amount of fat especially Omega 3 fatty acids in particular DHA (docosahexaenoic acid). In studies DHA levels determined levels of brain activity and cognitive function and is thought to be essential for the growth and functional development of the brain in babies. This ability is not limited to young humans as it is vital that this brain activity and function is maintained into old age. Including Omega 3 fatty acids in our diet therefore may well decrease our risk of developing degenerative brain diseases such as Alzheimer's.

Carrying additional weight can certainly contribute to strain on the heart muscle and the salmon has a rather unusual property that whilst yet unproven may help in weight loss.

There is a protein that is released when we begin to eat called amylin. This protein travels to the brain where it is measured and the brain then decides when we have eaten sufficient food and should stop eating. Unfortunately we have got very adept at overriding this message from the brain and consequently we tend to eat more than we actually need leading to weight gain.

The salmon produces a hormone called calcitonin, which has the same effect on animals as amylin does in humans. There is no conclusive proof but it is felt that this hormone when eaten might result in us consuming less food.

The other possible weight loss property of salmon is Chondroiton sulphate. Chondroiton is often used in conjunction with Glucosamine as a joint repair preparation but in this case the Chondroiton which is found in the nose of the salmon appears to have fat blocking capabilities. It appears to work in two ways by reducing the amount of fat absorbed into the intestines and then preventing any fat that has been absorbed from being stored in the cells. This will require a great deal more research but could be an interesting property in the fight against obesity.

As we get older the risk of bone fractures increases with many women particularly suffering from hip joint disease after menopause. Omega 3 may be instrumental in decreasing bone loss and therefore osteoporosis.

Our immune system is working ceaselessly against the constant onslaught of bacteria and viruses and on the whole if we have a healthy diet containing plenty of antioxidant rich foods our defence system keeps us safe. However, from time to time something slips through and then we need to know that all the complex mechanisms of the immune system are functioning perfectly.

Salmon is high in selenium, which is a very important trace mineral that activates an antioxidant enzyme called gluthatione peroxidase, which may help protect the body from cancer. It is vital for immune system function and may help prevent prostate cancer in particular.

Overall the salmon contains many nutrients in the flesh and also in parts of the fish such as bone that is often included in canned fish. It is an excellent source of calcium, magnesium, iron, iodine, manganese, copper, phosphorus and zinc, some of which are of particular benefit for the cardiovascular system and the heart.

Apart from its role in the formation of teeth and bones calcium is also required for blood clotting, transmission of signals in nerve cells and muscle contractions. There is some indication that higher calcium intake protects against cardiovascular disease particularly in women.

The main function of iron is in haemoglobin, which is the oxygen-carrying component of blood. When someone is iron deficient they suffer extreme fatigue because they are being starved of oxygen and the major organs of the body such as the heart also become deprived of this life essential element.

Salmon is very versatile and provided it is from a healthy source and not from poorly maintained fish farms it can be eaten two to three times a week served hot or cold with plenty of fresh vegetables and salads. It is particularly delicious served chilled with a spinach salad and new potatoes.

Turkey

Many people just associate turkey with Christmas or Thanksgiving in the USA but in fact as far as a protein in meat form goes, Turkey is actually packed full of nutrients and is an excellent all round food.

The wild turkey Meleagris gallopa (something to do with difficulty in catching it I think) is native to North America. The bird was imported into Europe in the early part of the 16th century by the Spaniards via Turkey (the country). It eventually was given its Latin name in the 18th century but the original name turkey stuck. The North Americans called it 'peru 'for some obscure reason, as it does not seem to have any connection with that country.

The Native American Indian used the turkey as a staple of their diet. They introduced it to starving pilgrims along with their native plants and seeds including corn and squash. The pilgrims were so grateful they celebrated the first Thanksgiving in 1621 where their short-lived American Indian friends were guests of honour.

Why Is Turkey Good for You?

Turkey is first and foremost a lean source of protein – 4 oz gives you 65% of your daily protein requirement and has about half the amount of saturated fat that red meat does.

We are protein – we need it to repair ourselves – a bit like the bionic man we take animal and vegetable protein, add some amino acids and rearrange the nitrogen from the mix to repair or make parts of our body. Don't forget we are meat – and a savoury delicacy still in certain parts of the world.

Turkey is very high in methionine, which is an essential amino acid that ensures that any protein that we eat is completely used. This makes sure that we get the maximum benefit from the turkey that we eat. This is particularly important if we find it difficult to digest food as we get older.

Turkey is very high in the amino acid tryptophan so it stimulates the B3 vitamin niacin into producing serotonin the neurotransmitter than not only has a calming effect and helps depression but also helps us sleep and feel good. Turkey is very high in Selenium, which is a trace mineral that is fundamental to our general health. It is involved in thyroid hormone metabolism – antioxidant defence systems and our immune system health – many studies into this mineral are revealing its positive effect on cancers. As an antioxidant it encourages DNA to repair cells and damaged cells to self-destruct.

Turkey is richer in calcium than any other meat and has over twice the calcium than chicken or beef. It also contains B6, which is extremely important for blood cell health.

It is also high in phosphorus, which is a fundamental need for bone and teeth formation and the production of red blood cells. Phosphorus is also part of the chemical energy store in each cell and in DNA so is vital for cell health. One of the things to watch for however with phosphorus is that it you eat a great many processed foods you will find that they are far too high in the mineral and can cause an imbalance with other minerals.

So Turkey is low fat, ½ in fact than even chicken, low in cholesterol, sodium and calories. Finally it is also called a short fibre meat which means that it is very easily digestible for any age group.

Seeds and Nuts

The following seeds are one of nature's male protectors and if every man ate a handful a day from childhood I am convinced there would be a great deal less prostate enlargement and cancer in middle age.

Pumpkin Seeds

When you look at a handful of pumpkinseeds it is very hard to imagine that each flat dark green 'pepita' is packed full of nutrients. Normally eaten roasted these nutty seeds contain protein, fibre, iron, copper, magnesium, manganese and phosphorus, all nutrients that we have covered in detail during the book. They also contain trace amounts of calcium, potassium, zinc, selenium, folate and B3 as well as Linolenic acid a property that prevents hardening of the arteries and amino acids Arginine and glutamic acid.

As with many of our natural remedies, pumpkin and their seeds played a vital role in the diet and health of the American Indian. Not only were they used for male health but also for urinary tract infections and in China they are regarded as a remedy for depression probably due to the presence of good levels of tryptophan and B3.

As with the melon, cucumber and squash the pumpkin belongs to the gourd or Cucurbitaceae family but pumpkin seeds are the most adaptable for consumption in their own right.

Pumpkin Seeds And Prostate Health

The reputation enjoyed by pumpkinseeds may be thousands of years in the making but modern research is backing the long held health claims.

It is thought that the oil containing cucurbitacins in the seeds may reduce the hormonal changes from testosterone to dihydrotestosterone that damages and increases the number of prostate cells that results in an enlarged prostate. It is also thought that they may well reduce the risk of developing prostate cancer.

Zinc in the seeds is also an important mineral as it helps to maintain semen volume and health as well as adequate levels of testosterone necessary for a healthy sex drive. The prostate gland actually contains the highest concentration of zinc in the body and certainly foods containing zinc may relieve symptoms of an enlarged prostate.

Apart from its effect on cholesterol it is thought that the Linolenic acid in pumpkinseeds may also improve urine flow among men with enlarged prostate glands.

The selenium in the seeds has many functions in the body but importantly in the case of the male reproductive system it is also believed to improve sperm motility and mobility. It is interesting that nearly 50% of a man's selenium is found in his testes and it is lost through ejaculation in the semen. Selenium also may protect against enlargement of the prostate as well as reduce damage to the cells that might develop into prostate cancer.

As an antioxidant, selenium may prevent oxidative damage to fats, vitamins, hormones and enzymes involved in normal prostate functioning.

Bone Health

Zinc in the seeds is also an important mineral that promotes bone density an often overlooked factor as men get older. It is often assumed that it is post menopausal women who are most at risk of hip fractures but in fact nearly a third of these fractures are suffered by men. Declining hormone levels effect men as they reach their fifties and sixties and osteoporosis of the hip and spine are becoming more common as our modern lifestyle results in nutritional deficiencies.

Cholesterol

Another side effect of modern life is the increasing levels of cholesterol in our bloodstream. Although 80% of our cholesterol is manufactured by our livers, if we consume high amounts of saturated fat in our diet we end up with far more than our overworked systems can cope with and process. It then is subjected to free radical damage and forms plaque in the arteries, blocking them and resulting in high blood pressure and ultimately heart disease.

As in the herb saw palmetto, phytosterols in pumpkin seeds actively work to reduce the levels of cholesterol in our bloodstream and eating a handful every day is much healthier in my opinion than eating the very expensive and hydrogenated alternative spreads to butter currently touted in our supermarkets. This applies to sesame seeds, which has the highest phytosterol content as well as unsalted pistachios and sunflower seeds.

Other Health Benefits

In addition to prostate, bone and the health of our arteries, eating pumpkinseeds may well help reduce the inflammatory diseases such as arthritis. In recent studies it was shown that not only did pumpkin seeds work as well as some prescribed medication but it did not have the unwelcome side effects and long term potential to further damage the lining of the joints.

Buying And Storing Pumpkin Seeds

It is not always a good idea to buy your seeds in bulk, as you want them to be as fresh as possible. Ensure that there is no damp in the packet and smell the seeds to detect any musty smell. They are best kept in an airtight container in the refrigerator and eat within a few weeks.

They are delicious eaten on their own as a snack during the day but also add a wonderful rich nutty flavour to salads or on roasted vegetables. If you make homemade burgers add a small handful to the meat mix before cooking and it will add a whole new dimension to the meal.

Sunflower Seeds

The sight of sunflowers as you drive through France on the way to England has always typified the weather and lifestyle of Mediterranean countries. They are one of my favourite flowers and I used one as a logo for my business in Ireland.

The seeds are a fantastic powerhouse of nutrients and including them in your healthy eating programme will only do you good.

Where Did Sunflowers Originate From?

It is believed that they originate from Mexico and Peru and they have been cultivated for around 5000 years, which is incredible. Indian

Americans have used the seeds to eat and the oil for that length of time and they also used the leaves, roots and stems for medicine and dyes. Powdered dry seeds have been used for centuries as a remedy for bronchitis, laryngitis, tonsillitis, influenza and coughs. It was even believed that growing the plant in your garden prevented you getting flu's and colds.

It actually was valued for its beauty as well as its food value. The Spanish explorers bought back seeds from South America and after being grown in Spain its use spread into France and into the rest of Europe. Russian and Eastern Europe have used it as an oilseed crop since the 18th century and the first commercial production of the oil was in 1830. Apart from South America, Spain, France and Russia, China is also a large commercial producer.

The larger seeds are used for eating and the smaller ones for the oil industry.

What About the Nutritional Properties?

Sunflower seeds are very high in Vitamin E, B1 and have healthy amounts of B-complex vitamins, manganese, magnesium, copper, tryptophan, selenium, phosphorus and Folate. One of their great benefits is the amount of protein that they contain along with essential fatty acids.

Of particular benefit are the high levels of Vitamin E, magnesium and selenium full details of which you can find in the chapter on essential nutrients.

What About the High Fat Content of Sunflower Seeds?

Actually Sunflower seeds contain what we term good fat in the form of essential fatty acids.

Essential fatty acids are very important to us, because they regulate oxygen use in the cells, are needed for healthy glandular function and increase levels of energy. Additionally they can alleviate allergies, symptoms of PMS, help lower LDL (lousy cholesterol) and raise HDL (healthy cholesterol), lower blood pressure, and they can lubricate joints and relieve the symptoms of arthritis.

So What Problems Could Eating Sunflower Seeds Help Prevent or Ease the Symptoms Of?

Apart from the anti-inflammatory effect on arthritis the high content of Vitamin E will also help prevent degenerative disease in the joints and the brain and lungs. Vitamin E is also essential for women going through the menopause as it can help with some of the more distressing symptoms such as hot flushes.

As an antioxidant it prevents free radical damage and this applies to cholesterol as well. When cholesterol is oxidised it becomes unstable and forms plaque on the walls of the arteries. This in turn narrows the artery restricting blood flow and allowing clots to form.

The magnesium in sunflower seeds not only helps regulate the flow of calcium between blood and bone but also helps keep our nervous and muscular system healthy. Spasms are extremely painful including those that are part of the symptoms of a heart attack; magnesium helps prevent this happening. Magnesium has also been found to be helpful in Asthma and reducing migraine headaches as it works like Vitamin E in an inflammatory capacity.

Selenium has long been regarded as a possible preventative for cancer. We need to detox our bodies naturally every day of the harmful toxins we have taken in through our skin, by breathing and in our food. The liver is home to many very powerful antioxidant enzymes specifically designed to get rid of toxic waste, one of which is Glutathione peroxidase. Selenium is very important in the manufacture of this enzyme and may be why it is so powerful as an anti-cancer agent. This may be explained because it is an antioxidant that not only encourages cells to repair themselves but also persuades cancerous cells to self-destruct.

What About Different Ways of Eating Sunflower Seeds?

The best way is to use them for snacks or to throw into your salads.

A very powerful but tasty way to eat your seeds and nuts is to make your own mix from pumpkinseeds, sunflower seeds and walnuts. A handful once a day will provide you with all the above nutrients, as they are all packed with them.

I love walnuts and seeds in my salads and you can grind the seeds up and use in sauces for your meat, fish and chicken.

You can also add to a homemade muesli mix.

Walnuts

Evidence of walnut consumption was dug up literally in Southwest France during excavation on Neolithic archaeological sites dating back over 8000 years. It appears that there were walnut groves in the hanging gardens of Babylon and in Greek mythology the walnut was highly revered and temples built to honour it.

The Latin name for the tree, Juglans Regia, comes from the Roman civilisation where it was called Jove Glans or the Royal nut of Jove. The nut and the oil have been used since ancient times both as a food and for dyeing wool and are now worldwide commodities.

Walnuts are very versatile – chopped up on savoury or sweet dishes or used as a snack between meals they give you a very healthy nutritional punch. Omega 3 fatty acids are a special type of protective fat rather than harmful fat and it is something that the body does not produce itself. – 14 half walnuts provides you with over 90% of your daily requirement and if you look at the health reasons for taking Omega 3 you will understand how very important this small handful of nuts is.

Omega 3 is known to help protect us from cardiovascular problems, improve brain function, help with inflammatory diseases such as asthma and arthritis and in skin diseases such as eczema and psoriasis. Walnuts also contain an antioxidant called ellagic acid, which boosts the immune system and protects against cancer.

The Most Important Benefit of Walnuts

For anyone who suffers from elevated LDL (lousy cholesterol) levels in their bloodstream eating walnuts is definitely helpful. It is one of those rare occasions when claims that certain foods can help a condition are permissible. In the case of walnuts the FDA in America were sufficiently convinced by scientific research into the benefits of the nuts in lowering cholesterol that they allowed the health claim to be advertised on products containing the nut or the oil. This is down to the excellent levels of Omega 3 in the nuts, which contain the highest amount in 1 oz compared to other nuts (2.5 gm of Omega 3 against 0.5 gm in other nuts)

Omega 3 helps prevent erratic heart rhythms and because the LDL is lowered which causes platelets to clot, the risk of strokes is also reduced.

Omega 3 works on our brain function because our brains are actually 60% structural fat and needs to be supported in our diet by specific Omega 3 fats like those in walnuts, flaxseeds and cold water fish like salmon. Part of the reason is that the cell membranes that everything has to pass through are mainly fat; Omega 3 is very flexible and fluid and can pass easily through the cell membrane taking other nutrients with it at the same time. This increases the cell uptake of nutrients making them more effective.

Studies of Omega 3 deficiency have highlighted some worrying trends. One of the most concerning is the evidence of depression in children. It has also been linked to hyperactivity, behavioural problems such as tantrums and learning difficulties. This deficiency is on the increase particularly in the United States, which means the UK won't be far behind.

Other Beneficial Nutrients in Walnuts

There are several other good reasons to include walnuts in your diet and they make a healthy addition to your daily diet as they include manganese, copper, Vitamin B6 and Tryptophan.

A portion of 9 walnut halves per day will therefore help protect the health of your skin, bone, cartilage. It will provide you with antioxidants, help synthesise some hormones and blood cells, produce collagen and assist in the formation of several neurotransmitters that regulate mood. The B6 will help lower the homocysteine levels in your blood which is linked to heart disease, osteoporosis and Alzheimer's disease and will help the release of carbohydrates stored in the liver and muscles for energy.

That is quite a nutritional punch for one small handful of nuts.

Extras to Include on a Daily Basis

Green Tea

All true teas – not herbal tisanes or infusions – are made from the Camellia Sinensis. These plants grow in warm climates with the very best teas coming from the highest altitudes – at that level the plant leaves are slower to mature and this means that they have a much richer flavour. Although the plants all come from the same strain – Camellia Sinensis – different growing conditions such as altitude, climate and soil will affect the flavour of the tea.

It is when the processing takes place that the difference appears between black and green teas. There is in fact another tea in the middle of these two, which is a greenish brown colour and is called oolong tea.

Green tea is the least processed of the three and therefore retains nearly all its nutritional content. One particular antioxidant which is called a Catechin (epigallocatechin-3-gallate EGCG for short) is believed to be responsible for the health benefits linked to green tea. Green tea is derived after the tealeaves have been gently steamed until they are soft, but have not fermented or changed colour. They are then rolled – spread out and fired which is either dried with hot air or fried in a wok until they are crisp. When you add boiling water to the leaves you get a pale yellowy green colour liquid.

Black tea on the other hand is first spread out on racks and withered with hot air – this removes about a third of their moisture and makes them soft. Then they are rolled which breaks the cell walls and releases juices. They are then laid out again in a high humidity environment to encourage the juice to ferment. The leaves turn a dark copper colour and are then fired turning the leaves black. This gives your tea its dark brown colour when you add boiling water to it.

Oolong tea is partially fermented which means it comes half way between the green and the black.

So *Green Tea Has More Antioxidants*

What Are its Main Health Benefits?

As with any food or supplement it is important not too over emphasis the health properties but in this case there is some compelling evidence to suggest that Green Tea has many benefits that could be effective in many different areas.

I talked about EGCG the flavanoid antioxidant, which is left in the green tea, and this is what researchers believe may be the secret to its health benefits. Because green tea is so widely drunk, mostly in Asian countries where dairy products are not used to flavour the tea – most of the early research was carried out in China and Japan. One of the diseases that has been studied is Coronary artery disease – there are indications that the antioxidant in green tea inhibits the enzymes that produce free radicals in the lining of the arteries. It has been shown to lower the LDL which if you remember is "lousy" cholesterol and improving the ratio to HDL Healthy cholesterol.

Drinking green team may help with stroke prevention because is thins the blood preventing blood clots from forming and travelling around the body. Eating a high fat diet can produce compounds in the blood that encourage platelets to clump together forming the clot. Not only that, it seems it may protect the cells in the heart muscle following damage so anyone recovering from a heart attack would find it a good tea to drink.

Researchers found that stroke victims who drank green tea were less likely to suffer any further damage and their brain cells were less likely to die off following an episode.

All of the above is linked to Green Tea's ability to thin the blood, therefore the flow is unrestricted and people are less likely to suffer from high blood pressure.

One of the largest areas of research is in Green Tea's possible protection against cancer. Obviously this is down to this incredible anti-oxidant EGCG but studies have also shown that apart from triggering cell suicide in cancer cells, apparently it might also inhibit the development of new blood vessels. Cancer like any parasite has an enormous appetite and the only way this can be catered for is for the body to produce new blood vessels in the form of a tumour. By inhibiting this, the green tea is effectively starving the cancer and it therefore dies.

What is even more interesting is that green tea has been shown to inhibit the growth of genetic cancerous cells such as those in breast cancer. Again it is this antioxidant's way of working that is so effective – it simply damages the rogue cells so much that it triggers a self-destruct mechanism that kills the cancer. The cancers that they have studied include Prostate, Ovarian, Breast and brain tumours in children. Colon, lung cancers have responded well and Green tea has been shown to improve the efficiency of cancer drugs while at the same time lessening their side effects.

Other diseases that have come under the microscope are diabetes, kidney disease, osteoporosis, gum disease, liver damage, Alzheimer's and Parkinson's disease. Epilepsy and green tea together are being researched because of the possible lessening effect of seizures in patients who drink it.

It has been shown to be anti-inflammatory which means that diseases such as rheumatoid arthritis may benefit – either from severity of the symptoms or preventing all together. Bacterial infections from tooth decay to intestinal problems such as Candida – where green tea catechins encourage a more acid environment that kills off the bad bacteria.

Viruses do not seem to like green tea and apparently it stops the virus from replicating which might be interesting for some diseases such as HIV where inhibiting replication is critical to prevent the disease from developing.

For example Japan where there is virtually only green tea consumption, they have a very low incidence of Alzheimer's, compared to western countries. However, Japanese living in the USA have 2.5 times the incidence of Alzheimer's of those living in Japan – In Japan people sip green tea all day – not so in the western environment or for 2nd and 3rd generation Japanese living in the USA. This particular health benefit has a knock-on effect on ageing as the cells are protected throughout the body for much longer.

The good news for anyone who is looking to lose weight is that Green tea has a thermogenic or fat burning effect on cells,

If you find it difficult to swap your current cup of breakfast tea with milk, try Green Tea with a slice of lemon, orange or lime. There are flavoured varieties on the market but as always it is better to avoid the over processed and add your own flavourings. It does have a distinctive taste but after a few cups of this nutritious tea you will enjoy adding it to your daily routine.

Honey

I doubt that there are many people today who are not aware of the health risks in consuming too much sugar rich food. Diabetes is on the increase, especially in children and along with obesity is likely to be one of the top causes of premature death within a few years.

To my mind the insidious inclusion of sugars in processed foods and equally as bad the introduction of toxic artificial sweeteners is one of the reasons for increased levels of cancer and degenerative diseases such as arthritis and Alzheimer's disease. We are becoming nutritionally deficient as we become more and more reliant on convenience and junk food laden with fats and sugars.

Honey is the exception and I encourage even my clients with Candida Albicans and Diabetes to use it as a healthy alternative to sugar or artificial sweeteners.

For thousands of years it has been used both as a nutritious addition to diet and as an effective medicine and the oldest reference to this delicacy dates back to 5500 BC. At that time Lower Egypt was actually called Bee Land while the Upper Egypt was called Reed Land. By 2500 BC bee keeping was well established and a thriving trade existed between Egypt and India where honey became associated with religious rites.

Apparently 110 large pots of honey was equivalent to one donkey or ox. Babylonian and Sumerian clay tablets describe honey's use as a medicine some of which included powdered bees and was considered a cure for bladder stones and dropsy. In all over half of the documented remedies recognised from these periods in our history were based on honey.

At first honey was treasured, due to not only its sweet taste but also its rarity. It was considered to be a divine substance and therefore it played a substantial role in many ancient people's rites and ceremonies. Apart from anointing the dead, jars of honey were sent into the next world to nourish the deceased and in some civilisations honey took on mythical and magical properties.

The Aztecs and Mayan cultures of South America kept colonies of native bees for their honey and wax, mainly for use as medicine.

Sometime in the 16th or 17th century settlers brought European bees into the Americas and honey became more available to everyone.

It is considered to be very pure and therefore used in marriage rites around the world including in our own expression of honeymoon as it promoted fertility and was thought to act as an aphrodisiac.

If all that is not enough to tempt you to use honey on a daily basis then some of the health benefits of honey may be able to persuade you.

Health Benefits of Honey

Having given honey such a wonderful lead in I now have to put in a proviso and that is that not all honey is created equal.

Bees make honey for their own nourishment from the nectar collected from flowers and the enzymes in their saliva. They carry the honey back to the hive where it is deposited in the cells in the walls where it dries out and forms that consistency that we are familiar with.

The quality and medicinal qualities of honey are very dependent on the plants that the bees producing that honey have had access to. Most of the commercially available honey originates from bees feeding on clovers, heather and acacia plants but there are some wonderful flavours available from bees with access to herb plants such as thyme and lavender.

Unfortunately in the processing of wild honey to the commercially acceptable product you find on most supermarket shelves, many of the nutrients can be lost.

One honey in particular that is a very valuable anti-bacterial agent is Propolis, the glue that bees use to seal the hive and protect the contents. This is usually present in small amounts if wild honey but is lost in processing unless it is specifically included. You can buy Propolis honey but it can be a little more expensive but worth it.

One of the best honeys in the world comes from New Zealand and is called Manuka honey and because of its reputation for healing it is very heavily tested and regulated to maintain its high standards.

Active Manuka honey is used both internally and externally to treat a number of medical conditions and research is being conducted to legitimise the claims that are made of its effectiveness which show a great deal of promise. Currently it may help prevent stomach ulcers, poor digestion, gastritis, Helicobacter Pylori (H.Pylori), skin ulcers, sore throats, skin infections, boost immune system and energy levels. It is thought that it might even work effectively against MRSA, which would be very interesting.

If you are eating honey then do buy locally and if possible from source. Visit the beekeeper and you should see someone in glowing health, which will be a testament to the quality of his bees and honey. We have bee farms near where we live in Madrid and they are miles from pollution and surrounded by wild plants of every variety in the hills.

Internal Health Benefits

Good quality raw honey is anti-bacterial, anti-viral and anti-fungal. It is also an amazing energy source and certainly Greek athletes used both honey and figs to enhance their performance on the track. Modern researchers conducted a study using athletes, some of which were given a honey, some sugar and some maltodextrin as the carbohydrate source. The athletes who were given the honey maintained a steady blood sugar level throughout the two hour training session and their recovery times was much better than those athletes on the alternative energy sources.

For anyone suffering from diabetes, finding a sweetener that does not affect blood sugar levels dramatically is vitally important and honey would appear to raise levels far less than any other refined alternative. However, this still does not mean that a diabetic can eat honey freely but it does mean that breakfast porridge and cups of tea can benefit from a little sweetness if it is required.

It has also been found that natural honey rather than processed honey can help reduce cholesterol levels, homocysteine levels and increases the level of HDL (healthy cholesterol) helping to prevent heart disease.

Honey's healing properties are beneficial for stomach ulcers, sore throats and intestinal damage with a balancing effect on intestinal bacteria. This includes Candida Albicans, which goes against most therapists' philosophy of eliminating all sweeteners from a sufferer's diet. All my clients have switched to honey in their programmes and it seems to not only help in the recovery but also provides a small element of sweetness to satisfy cravings.

It has been found that taking natural honey on a daily basis raises blood levels of the protective antioxidant compounds that we need to prevent disease and to heal ourselves. Admittedly the subjects in the study that confirmed this consumed four tablespoons of buckwheat honey per day which would grate on even my sweet tooth. I do believe as you know in the accumulative effect and therefore over a period of time taking a teaspoon or so of honey per day on food or in drinks should benefit you in the long term.

External Health Benefits

As with ulcers internally, honey is excellent for external wound healing. Honey absorbs water in the wound inhibiting the growth of bacteria and fungi. Also honey contains glucose oxidase that when mixed with water produces hydrogen peroxide which is a mild antiseptic. There are also specific enzymes in honey, particularly Manuka honey that appear to speed up the healing process in combination with the common antioxidant properties.

Do spend that little bit extra for Propolis or Manuka honey to obtain the most health benefits but also try and source your honey from a local beekeeper who can show you the variety and quality of the flowers available to his bees.

Olive Oil

As you will have seen in the nutrients section of the book essential fatty acids (EFA's) are vital for most areas of our health including our sexual health.

Olive oil contains these EFA's in abundance and using it as an alternative to particularly the hydrogenated fats in processes margarines and oils is essential. Lowering your cholesterol is one of the main objectives in changing your current lifestyle and using olive oil both for cooking and on salads will help you do so.

Olive oil is also an excellent source of Vitamin E and phenols.

The Benefits of Olive Oil

Extra virgin olive oil which is from the first pressing of the olives is the best oil to use as it contains higher levels of nutrients, particularly Vitamin E and phenols above. Recent research into the reasons why Olive oil so extensively used in Mediterranean diets is so healthy has thrown up some interesting results.

In a human trial it was found that polyphenol rich olive oil included in the diet improved the health of blood vessels which was not the case for another group of volunteers that included oil in their diet with the phenols removed. Obviously the healthier the blood vessels the more effective the entire circulatory system. It appears that the particular part of the blood vessel that is affected is the endothelium or inner lining of the blood vessels. The endothelium determines the interactions between the blood vessels and the immune, coagulation and endocrine systems. If the endothelium is not functioning correctly it can lead to calcification within the arteries and increased risk of heart disease and strokes. Another function of the endothelium is the release of vasodilators (increasing size of blood vessel) such as Nitric Oxide and vasoconstrictors (decreasing size of blood vessels) such as thromboxane and prostaglandin. Like any system in the body balance or homeostasis is required to ensure that blood pressure is regulated and the phenols in olive oil ensure that sufficient nitric oxide is produced to keep the arteries open and blood flowing.

Other Research Areas

Until now it has been difficult to isolate which component of this very nutrient rich oil was responsible for the health of Mediterranean populations. Recently however in America they have identified a previously unknown chemical that they have called oleocanthal that appears to have an extremely effective anti-inflammatory action. They have compared it favourably with over the counter pain relievers for inflammatory conditions such as ibuprofen. This is great news for sufferers of inflammatory diseases such as arthritis.

Other Benefits of Olive Oil

Olive oil is very well tolerated by the digestive system and is therefore beneficial for stomach ulcers and gastritis. The oil activates the secretion of bile and pancreatic hormones much more effectively than prescribed medication and therefore lowers the incidence of gallstone formation.

Two tablespoons of a day has been shown to lower oxidation of LDL (lousy cholesterol) in the blood whilst raising antioxidant levels such as Vitamin E.

It is suggested that including olive oil in your diet may also help prevent colon cancer and this provides an alternative to patients who are vegetarian and do not wish to include fish oils in their diet.

Including extra virgin olive oil every day in your diet is likely to protect you from diseases such as atherosclerosis, diabetes, asthma, breast cancer and arthritis.

The Best Oil to Buy

As I have always said the less processed a food is the better and olive oil is no exception. On the shelf you will find at least four different grades of oil.

- Extra Virgin which is the best, least processed and most nutritional and comes from the first pressing. This should be your first choice and used for all cooking and dressings during your detox period.
- Virgin is from the second pressing and should be your second choice.
- Pure undergoes some processing such as filtering and refining and is a lesser grade oil.
- Extra Light – has undergone considerable processing and only retains a small amount of nutrients or even olive taste. It is not officially classified as an olive oil and it was produced more for the "diet" culture than for taste or nutrition.

Storing Olive Oil

Olive oil degrades in light and should be kept cook and tightly sealed. If it is exposed to air oxygen will turn it rancid. It is also better kept in a cupboard away from natural light and the best containers are ceramic jugs rather than glass or plastic bottles.

How to Use Olive Oil

Use extra virgin olive oil in casseroles and soups to add flavour. It is better to use in its natural state on salads, bread and over steamed vegetables or rice.

Action Plan

I told you at the beginning of this book that this was not an instant solution to either your current health problems or your sexual dysfunction.

What I would ask is that you give yourself six weeks to show me that I am wrong. Begin the Healthy Eating Plan for life exactly and then decide for yourself if being slimmer, fitter more energetic and healthier has not made a difference in other areas of your life such as your sex drive and performance.

At the very least if you have been monitoring your blood pressure, cholesterol and blood sugar then you should see an improvement in all these areas which will reduce your risk of developing more serious diseases such as diabetes or heart failure.

If you do not feel better then of course there is always the 'little blue pill' but I hope that you will see enough of an improvement that you will want to keep going until this way of living and eating is not just a six week diet but a change for life. Also please do not keep the good news to yourself – pass the message on to every man that you meet even if they do not feel that they are risk of disease or sexual dysfunction – the earlier that you start taking care of yourself the longer your active sex life.

It may not be macho to talk about eating healthily in the pub or the locker room but at the end of the day we only have one life and it is for living. It is not for sitting watching life happening to other people on the television or dreaming of your youth. It is about making the most of the here and now and loving every minute.

Like any addict you will find that at first it will be hard to give up certain behaviours and habits. Remember you have taken forty or fifty years to get to this point, is four weeks or ten weeks really that much of a challenge when there could be so many rewards at the end of it.

It is in *your* hands, and only you can make the decision.

Here it comes – the beginning of the rest of your life …

The Cronin Nutritional Healthy Eating Plan for Life (and Possibly a Great Sex Life)

Over the last fifteen years I have developed the original eating programme that I designed to help me get fit, into an easy to follow, healthy and effective way to lose weight. But weight is not just the only issue when we talk about diets. We as a living organism have a requirement for a specific combination of nutrients. Our bodies are very sophisticated and employ complex mechanisms to extract, utilise and combine nutrients to achieve optimum health. Like any good recipe we need to provide our bodies with the basic ingredients and the correct environment for this to happen. I believe that it is not the one huge change that you make to your lifestyle that creates improvements to your health and weight but the 101 small changes that make the biggest difference. Even if you are currently following a reasonably healthy lifestyle, you do need to review your strategies on a regular basis as you age or your life changes pace. What you are able to eat at twenty years old or even thirty-five is different when you get into your 40's and 50's.

This plan can be adapted for your age, gender and activity level and by following the basic rules you will find over a period of weeks and months that you are leaner and healthier than you have ever been before.

At this stage it is more important to get into the good habits and discard your bad habits than it is to count calories. However it is as important to take in sufficient calories as it is to not take in too many. If you lose weight too quickly you are in danger of losing muscle. Your body as we have already stated needs a complex cocktail of nutrients to function and to survive. If you do not feed your body with the raw ingredients it has to go somewhere to find them and that is your storage system in your muscles and your bones. Apart from eroding bone and lean muscle mass you will be reducing your body's requirement for fuel and will therefore affect your metabolism.

Muscle burns fuel more efficiently and if you lose that muscle your body will store any excess as fat. This is why we tend to put weight back on with extra pounds when we have been on a severely restricted diet. Starvation levels of dieting below a thousand calories have long term effects on your health and longevity. Osteoporosis is a very real danger to women and men who have persisted with low calorie and nutrient diets during their early years.

My recommendation is that men do not reduce their calories below 1800 calories per day when trying to lose weight. Of equal importance is that the food that you take in within that calorie range is nutrient packed and you will this is where the inclusion of nutrient rich superfoods in this programme is so essential.

The aim of this eating plan is also to reduce your risk of developing high blood pressure and cholesterol but also to reduce levels if they are already too high.

A Note For Those of You Who Do not Cook for Yourselves

A few years ago I was visited by the wife of one of my clients who was furious with me. She told me in no uncertain terms that she had been cooking three meals a day for her husband for the last 30 years and now he was coming home with a list of foods and meals that he was to eat instead. The husband in question had very high blood pressure, cholesterol and was about four stone overweight. His doctor had been trying to get him to lose weight and eat a healthy diet for five years.

This is going to require some diplomacy. It is very important that you do not go flying into the house brandishing this book and announce to your hard working wife that she needs to change the way she cooks for you.

As a woman I have to say that I would probably go off the deep end myself. I suggest that you sit down and discuss your health issues or your desire to prevent future problems and explain that you would like to make some minor changes to your diet. It would be even better if you suggest that perhaps you might help out with the shopping, preparation and cooking (washing up too is also a winner). This is going to mean changes not just for you but very possibly for the rest of your family too but I have usually found that a wife wants what is best for the man in her life and I am sure that you will find that she will be more than happy to help you make these changes.

The other bonus is that your wife if she is anything like me has been on constant body watch most of her life and the good news is that she can eat the same diet and perhaps enjoy some of the benefits.

Whilst it sounds a bit over the top to call what follows "rules" it is important that you follow them to ensure that you are getting enough food and fluids to be healthy and that you understand why you are following each one.

Rule 1: You Must Eat Breakfast

Everyone is to have breakfast, even if you say you are not a breakfast person and you should eat within an hour of getting up in the morning. Even if it is a fruit juice and some fruit salad with a tea or coffee you must eat something to kick start your metabolism and get your blood sugar to a level that will sustain your energy throughout the day. As you will see from the example menus I prefer a whole grain start to the day which will give you energy and sustain that energy throughout the morning.

Rule 2: You Must Eat at Least Six Times a Day

This is three moderate meals and 3 snacks. If you weigh more than 3 stone overweight you will have an additional snack a day and if you are over 5 stone overweight you will have an additional 2 snacks a day. Your body requires fuel on a continuous basis and will use and process these six meals without storing fat. Because the calories will be less than your body requires on a daily basis you will be using up more than you are taking in, resulting in weight loss.

This is probably the point that I should repeat my previous warnings about portion size. It is easy to justify eating a bit more if the food is healthy but we are not very good about being exact about the amount of calories in a particular ingredient of a meal let alone the whole meal.

A couple of guidelines for you

For some reason our human brains count in twos. When was the last time you had just one biscuit or one piece of toast or one drink.

It seems automatic to take one for later! Get into the habit of just having one sandwich for example rather than automatically making two that you feel obliged to eat.

It is not necessarily the piece of toast that is the problem or the medium sized jacket potato – it is the toppings that make the difference. A scrape of butter, a teaspoon of marmalade etc is all you need for the taste. And just because you are only having one piece of toast instead of two does not mean having the double ration of butter and marmalade.

If you are currently eating off a very large plate downsize. Take what you need and finish your plate. Leave for at least 10 minutes before you go back for more – that will give your stomach time to tell your brain you are full.

With carbohydrates, which are an essential part of your energy fuel, you need to think in terms of wholegrain or in vegetables and fruit. It is the grain carbohydrates which are the most calorific and I suggest that you use a coffee mug as a measure for a cooked portion of both.

Rule 3: You Must Drink at Least 2 Litres of Pure Water Per Day

Not all at once but throughout the day starting with a glass of water as soon as you wake up. You will be dehydrated after a nights sleep and you need to restore your mineral balance before you start the day. We cannot survive much longer than six minutes without air, six days without water or six weeks without food. That makes hydration your second highest priority for survival. The food you eat does effect your hydration. Salad foods particularly have high water content and even dry foods contain some too. However, we lose fluid through breathing, our skin and going to the toilet and that needs to be replaced. Anyone who tells you that you do not need to drink water at all is seriously affecting your health.

Rule 4: Whatever Alcohol You Are Currently Drinking You Must at Least Halve It

Alcohol is in our lives to a lesser or greater extent. We use it in celebration or when we are depressed, to reward ourselves, to put us in the mood or to fit in with our friends. Taken in moderation, alcohol still has a physical effect on our bodies. Certainly some has a mildly therapeutic effect but red grape juice has as many Bioflavonoids as red wine.

Our liver is the organ that takes the full brunt of any alcohol intake that we indulge in, and as the liver is such a vital organ in the elimination of toxins and waste, it is vital that it is protected throughout our lifetime. A healthy liver can determine much of our overall general health and longevity so respecting it makes very good sense.

Liver cirrhosis as a result of alcohol is one of the ten leading causes of death in the United States and I would assume on a similar level in parts of the UK. Excessive drinking can be responsible for altering brain activity affecting your concentration and reflexes. This is very evident in drink driving. Mild symptoms may be insomnia, heartburn and slightly raised blood pressure.

The more dangerous side effects however can be fatal. Alcohol can raise levels of triglycerides in the blood causing arterial and heart disease. It affects the levels of calcium in the body leading to osteoporosis. Obesity is very common with all of its complications and there are indications that there is a serious increase in the risks of many cancers including in the mouth, pharynx, larynx, oesophagus, liver and breast.

I am not intending to blackmail you into giving up alcohol, but like any toxin that we choose to take into our body, we should do so fully informed and not with our head stuck in the sand. We now are fully informed of the dangers of smoking and over the last few months there has been an emphasis on the dangers of excessive or binge drinking. Hopefully this will save lives over the next few years.

I don't expect anyone to give up alcohol altogether but you will notice an amazing difference in your energy levels and the way that you feel if you do. But at least by halving your intake you will see some benefit. Do think about this carefully however and if you can manage with just one glass of wine with your dinner each night that would be tremendous. Take a close look at how much you are actually consuming at present and multiply each glass of wine by 100 calories and see how these invisible calories are impacting not just your weight but your health. One half bottle of wine per night represents 36 lbs or 17 kilos in excess body fat a year. If you only need to lose 14 lbs or 6 kilos you can do that by reducing your intake to half.

Rule 5: Have a Little Protein With Each Meal

You don't have to eat 100 of grams of protein with every meal or snack. But one chicken breast – 5 oz of salmon – light cream cheese spread – semi skimmed milk – 1 oz of cheddar etc. included with and between meals will be affective. Give yourself a couple of meat free days per week and for example have a meal using half an avocado which is not only a good source of vitamins and minerals but also of healthy fat with a fresh green salad including broccoli and beans.

You will find the essential and non-essential amino acids that the body needs in a wide variety of plant based foods including lentils, peanuts, broad beans, kidney beans, pumpkin seeds, sunflower seeds, walnuts and vegetables.

We are made of protein and proteins are essential to the structure, function, and regulation of the body including the systems that produce hormones, enzymes, and antibodies. If you are considering becoming a vegetarian or you are already one then do make sure that you are taking in sufficient protein in your diet to satisfy your body's needs.

Clients who have come to me with various health problems have accused me of being anti-vegetarianism in the past. This is not the case. I am firmly against starvation diets, which is a different matter altogether. Most of the clients I have worked with who have chosen to give up animal products have done so without thought to the alternatives they needed to substitute to give them the essential nutrients required to be healthy. They have in some case simply reduced the amount of food and variety that they eat every day. It has been an emotional decision, not a considered one. You can have a wonderfully healthy diet without animal protein and if you need help in designing that programme contact a Nutritional therapist and get their assistance.

Rule 6: Make a Fresh Fruit Salad and Have at Least One Bowl Each Day

Fruit is a wonderful way to take in many of the vitamins and anti-oxidants that you need on a daily basis. In our supermarkets today there is an amazing array of European and tropical fruit that is fresh and tastes wonderful. Any fruit that you eat is a 'superfood' in my book. This is a very simple recipe but you can substitute any fruits that are your particular favourites. For dinner parties splash out on the more exotic fruits such as mango and papaya and serve with home made ice cream. Your guests will love it.

Use unsweetened apple juice and take 2 red apples, 2 large pears – half a melon – half a fresh pineapple – 2 large plums. Substitute your favourite fruit and alternate on a weekly basis so that you get plenty of variety.

Cut all the fruit up and store in a large airtight container in the fridge and this will last you at least three days – that is if you can keep the rest of the family out of it. However, just think how much good it will do them – especially if they eat this instead of a high sugar or fat snack.

If you don't like your fruit salad plain you can serve with live yoghurt.

Rules sound a little draconian but to be honest when it comes to your health you cannot afford to be half hearted. This applies to rule 7 of the plan and some of you might be quite shocked at my insistence that you either stop drinking or severely restrict your intake of canned soft drinks. I think that when you see the reasoning behind my concerns you will agree that it is unlikely that these drinks are actually doing you any good and in many cases maybe doing you harm.

Rule 7: Whatever Else You Drink, Do not Touch Diet Drinks or Canned Drinks and If You Do Restrict to Once or Twice a Week

I covered the downside to drinking fizzy drinks in the first part of the book. We are trying to reduce not just the sugars in processed food and drink but also all the additives that they contain.

Rule 8: Whatever Your Current Exercise Level Put More Energy Into It

You either love it or hate it but exercise is extremely important for the body. It not only tones our muscles, burns fat and builds healthy bone but it makes us feel great. Even if you drag yourself out of bed in the morning and groan at the thought of that cold and wet morning out there, you will feel invigorated at the end of your 30 minute brisk walk.

One of the areas that we don't concentrate enough on is our breathing. We need oxygen to survive but most of us do not breathe deeply enough to obtain the amount we need nor do we then get rid of all the waste from our bodies which is expelled every time we breathe out.

Walking every day briskly for 30 to 45 minutes will not only help you lose weight and tone your muscles but is also weight bearing. This improves both your bone density and the flexibility of your muscles, tendons and joints. Your heart will benefit as the oxygen rich blood is pushed through the arteries clearing blockages and taking the nutrients around the body. Your brain will benefit and you will feel very good about yourself. If you have not been exercising recently then start with a 20 minute walk at some stage during the day and the gradually build this up to 45 minutes. You can incorporate breathing exercises in the beginning that will help improve your internal health as well as build up your stamina.

Dancing, tennis, light weight training, golf and swimming can be integrated into your exercise programme and you need to put energy and commitment into the process to get the maximum benefit.

Do give yourself one or two days off though once a week, rest is also important to allow your body to recover and recharge itself. You need to be following the Healthy Eating Plan to ensure that you are getting the right level of calories and nutrients to enable you to exercise without using up all your reserves. Do not be tempted to starve yourself and work out too hard, as you will weaken both your immune system and cause long-term damage to your bones and organs.

Rule 9: Changing Habitual Eating Patterns

A normal chocolate bar a day for a year is 55 lbs or 25 kilos in body fat – a Danish pastry every morning with your coffee is 67 lbs per year or 31 kilos. Two digestive biscuits with your coffee each morning equates to 20 lbs per year. Just think about that before you reach for them. Do you need them every day? If you cut down to twice or three times a week you will be losing between 10 lbs and 34 lbs per year automatically. Take a look at your diet and you may find that there are one or two regular food items that you could reduce and lose weight easily and healthily.

Rule 10: Salt

Excess salt can cause raised blood pressure. When blood is over salty it retains fluids, which increases the volume in the arteries. This causes a rise in the pressure. The recommended amount of salt is 5 gm for women and 7 gm for men. However, a useful measure is one level teaspoon per day. Put a level teaspoon times the amount of people you are cooking for in a coffee cup or something similar and add pinches to your cooking and to taste on your meals. If you run out before the evening, then I am afraid that is it. If you must put salt on your food put on the side of the plate and only use when absolutely necessary. Read food labels on processed foods, and do not forget to check your mineral water. Multiply the sodium levels by 2.5 and see just how much salt you are drinking let alone eating.

You now have the basic rules of the eating plan and if you work with these you will find it both easy to stick to the programme in the long term and also ensure a successful outcome.

The Eating Plan

In the previous chapters I have outlined both the nutrients you need to be fit, healthy and sexy and some of the most important food groups to include daily. I hope that now you have a better understanding of the history and nutritional content of the most common everyday foods that you will also have a healthier respect for them and the affect on your body.

Make a list of all those foods and also any other fruits, vegetables, seeds and nuts that are your personal favourites and work them into the example menus that follow.

Remember that the aim is to keep your diet 80% natural and unprocessed and only 20% processed. A challenge to begin with but once you get into the swing of it you will be surprised at how salty, sweet and chemical you find processed sauces and dishes.

I have prepared a basic shopping list that you can add to as you discover new foods that are fresh and unprocessed that you can add to your diet as you wish. The only area to be a little careful is with your protein choices. The fat around a steak is very tasty and the temptation is to justify eating it because it is natural and unprocessed. Well you can also have too much of a good thing. Get into the habit of trimming most – not all – of the fat off your protein choices. You can still enjoy the taste whilst minimising the calories and the affect on your cholesterol levels.

Also on that note – however healthy the food it does have a calorie and fat value and if you are planning on losing weight then you need to factor that in. Counting calories is tedious but perhaps for the first few weeks you might find a calorie counter useful to get you accustomed to healthy portion sizes. You will find some very useful ones online. The other useful tool is a food diary that you keep for a week or two as this will highlight areas that perhaps you are being over indulgent. Nothing like seeing it in writing.

After the shopping list you will find some example menus for 14 days – this is only to stimulate your interest in variety. Eating the same things day after day might be time saving and less hassle but in fact you are more likely to stick to an eating programme if there is plenty of variety in it.

Shopping List

This weekly shopping list contains foods that are nutrient packed. Apart from the obvious fresh fruit and vegetables there are also specific foods that play a role in healing the body.

This list is not exhaustive but is designed to give you an idea of the foods that you need to include on a daily or regular basis to provide your body with the nutrients it needs to be healthy.

Fresh Fruit And Vegetables

You will need to have eight portions of vegetables per day. You will also be eating four portions of fruit either as part of a fruit salad or as a snack. Lemons will form one portion of fruit per day in the form of juice first thing in the morning. As you will be eating salads or steamed vegetables at lunch and dinner this is easy to achieve. A portion is two tablespoons of carrots and loose vegetables, one large potato, large tomato, and whole avocado.

Fluids

Start every morning with a cup of hot water and lemon juice- It will help alkalise your body and kick start your digestive system.

Unsweetened fresh pressed juices both vegetable and fruit. Supermarkets will usually have a selection available. If not buy unsweetened juice only products from the chill cabinet. They are more expensive but they have no colourants or preservatives. For example orange and carrot juice – smoothies that have no additives.

- Still mineral water
- Green Tea
- Peppermint tea
- Any organic detox tea
- Herbal teas – all fruits.

Vegetables

Again it is important that you have as much variety as possible. If you are making a Brown Rice Pilaf this is quite easy as you can steam 7 or 8 vegetables – use a portion of each with one portion of rice. Always have two dark green vegetables at least – broccoli and spinach etc. There is no problem in using good quality frozen vegetables that have been picked and frozen quickly.

- Asparagus
- Aubergine
- Avocado
- Broccoli
- Brussel sprouts
- Cabbage
- Carrots
- Cauliflower
- Celery
- Courgettes
- Cucumbers
- Garlic
- Green Beans
- Lettuce Rocket is best
- Leeks
- Mushrooms (shitake if possible. These have tremendous healing properties for cholesterol, blood pressure and blood sugar.)
- Olives
- Onions
- Parsnips
- Frozen Peas
- Potatoes
- Swedes
- Seeds and beans (freshly sprouted and found in the specialist green grocer section of supermarkets have the highest levels of nutrients designed to feed the growing plant. Very nutty and great on salads)
- Spinach
- Red Peppers
- Tomatoes
- Yams or Sweet Potatoes (excellent nutrients)

Fruit

A fresh fruit salad in a sealed container in the fridge will keep for a couple of days and is great with yoghurt. If you are going to work or on the move choose the less sugary varieties as they tend not to go off and make sure they are thoroughly washed. Bananas are a great travelling fruit.

- Apples – Crisp green.
- Apricots fresh or dried (if dried make sure without sulphates and only have one or two as concentrated sugar)
- Bananas
- Blueberries (expensive but only need a few in a fruit salad to give an antioxidant punch)
- Figs (the best source of alkaline forming foods that reduces acidity in the stomach and the blood)
- Kiwi (very high concentration of Vitamin C)
- Lemons (for fresh lemon juice each morning with hot water)
- Oranges
- Mango
- Melon
- Papaya
- Pears
- Pineapple (eaten freshly cut will help inflammation in joints due to high Bromelain content)
- Plums
- Raisins and sultanas to use with porridge to sweeten. Again only a dessertspoon as high in sugars.
- Strawberries

Nuts Seeds and Oils. (All Nuts Should Be Unsalted)

- Almonds
- Brazils
- Cashews (these can cause diarrhoea so only eat one or two at a time)
- Flaxseeds or Linseeds (organic can be found in some upmarket supermarkets but more usually in Health Food shops – a dessertspoon on porridge and salads provides both fibre and EFAs.)
- Pumpkinseeds – every man should be snacking on these for prostate health from 45 onwards.

- Sesame seeds
- Sunflower seeds
- Walnuts
- Extra Virgin Olive Oil. For cooking, salad dressings and for drizzling on potatoes etc.
- Flaxseed oil Use in dressings or drizzled on vegetables.
- Benecol or Flora spread

Grains
- Natural porridge oats (do not use instant porridge as it is loaded with everything else but nutrients) Health food sections of supermarkets
- Wheatgerm (very high in nutrients and fibre)
- Wholegrain cereals without additives if possible but definitely no sugar Weetabix, shredded wheat or similar
- Wholegrain rye crispbreads or multigrain (quite tasty without spread but with mashed banana and cinnamon.)
- Brown Rice
- Corn tortillas
- Home made Muesli (recipe in book)

Beans
If you really do not have time to prepare beans then buy the jars in the supermarket and rinse thoroughly before use.

- Chickpeas
- Kidney beans
- Cannellini Beans
- Soya (can buy frozen ones and use as vegetable)
- Lentils

Spices and Herbs
Use freely but in particular you will find the following useful.

- Basil
- Black Pepper
- Cayenne Pepper
- Oregano
- Paprika
- Pimiento

- Salt (no more than 1 level teaspoon per day for cooking and seasoning)
- Balsamic Vinegar (healthy and very tasty for salad dressings)
- Turmeric (great anti-oxidants – research showing curcumin in turmeric is anti-dementia, arthritis, cancer – generally great for chronic autoimmune)

Dairy Products

I prefer to use natural products rather than man made alternatives. Use semi-skimmed milk – eat cheese sparingly – try goat's cheese it is stronger and you need less. If you really feel you want to use the products that promise to reduce your cholesterol then go ahead but to be honest a drizzle of olive oil on your bread or potatoes is just as tasty.

Use olive oil instead of butter or margarine for vegetables.

Meat and Poultry

(Very necessary for the protein but in particular the B vitamins)
- Lean Beef – (once a week)
- Calves liver – (once a week ask at the meat counter)
- Chicken
- Lamb
- Ostrich
- Turkey
- Venison

Fish

Should never be breaded or battered. Grilled with olive oil and lemon juice.

- Cod
- Hake
- Halibut
- Monkfish
- Perch
- Salmon
- Sardines (fresh grilled with the bones excellent source of EFAs and Calcium)
- Sea Bass
- Swordfish

- Trout
- Tuna

Sweeteners

Please do not use any artificial sweeteners they contain chemicals that mimic the bodies reaction to sugar

- Honey (natural antibiotic and great for healing leaky gut caused by Candida)
- Dried Fruit (in moderation as this concentrated sugar the exception being apricots which are very powerful therapeutically)

Note

Feel free to buy any other fruit and vegetable that appeal to you. Also fish and lean cuts of meat as long as it is not processed. If you can buy organic meat then that would be best.

Fourteen-Day Example Menus

You now have the ingredients for your new healthy eating plan. How you put them together is down to you as long as you have three main meals and three snacks. To give you an idea of the different meals and snacks you could eat I have put together the following lists.

This fourteen day menu is intended as an example only and needs to be adjusted to your needs. You can have your main meal either at lunchtime or the evening but it is better for you to have your carbohydrates at lunchtime rather than later in the day as you are unlikely to use them up. However, if you eat around the 6.00–7.00 pm time and then are active in some form afterwards you are fine.

Here is a reminder of my "superfoods" list and it would be a good idea to include at least six of these every day.

Oranges, Oats, Green Tea, Bananas, Walnuts, Spinach, Broccoli, Onions, Salmon, Turkey, Brown Rice and Avocado

You will find most of the fruit juices in the smaller size in packs of six which will keep them fresh over the two week period and the portion size is about right. Go for unsweetened or pure juices that you have made yourself.

I have included some useful recipes at the back of the book to get you started but there are some wonderful cookery books on the market these days that are full of low fat, nutrient packed ideas for meals.

14 Breakfasts

1. Cranberry juice, corn tortilla, one scrambled egg, orange and green tea.
2. Apple juice, porridge with semi-skimmed milk and honey, apple and green tea.
3. Orange juice, bowl of rice crispies, banana and green tea

4. Grapefruit juice, weetabix, strawberries and green tea
5. Cranberry juice, poached egg on one slice of toast, orange and green tea.
6. Apple juice, porridge with honey, banana and green tea.
7. Fresh fruit salad with low fat yoghurt, piece of toast and marmalade with green tea.
8. Grapefruit juice, weetabix, berries and green tea
9. Cranberry juice, corn tortilla with two lean rashers of bacon, apple and green tea
10. Apple juice, porridge with raisins, orange and green tea
11. Orange juice, cornflakes with berries, green tea.
12. Grapefruit juice, rice crispies with banana and green tea.
13. Cranberry juice, beans on toast, apple and green tea.
14. Fresh fruit salad with low fat yoghurt, piece of toast and marmalade with green tea.

Main Meals

Some of the main meals can be prepared and then frozen. I do this with the stuffed peppers and it makes it quick and easy to microwave them when you get home from work.

It is important to have as much variety as possible in your meals so that you get the widest spread of nutrients. Try not to fall into the habit of having the same meal on the same day every week. When you are working it is hard to feel motivated to prepare a dinner from scratch every night but things like brown rice, mashed potato and pasta can all be prepared and then frozen. Vegetables too keep for at least four days in a sealed container in the refrigerator so make enough to store and then use as needed. Personally I eat three portions of fruit and five portions of vegetables at least per day and I often eat carrots or other green vegetables most nights of the week.

14 Main Meals

1. Roast lamb or cutlets, carrots with two dark green vegetables, jacket potato with drizzle of olive oil. Peppermint tea.
2. Spinach salad with tomato and cucumber, Turkey wrap (wholegrain) with peppers and onions and peppermint or green tea.
3. Stuffed peppers with brown rice tuna, onions and peppers. Raw vegetable salad and peppermint or green tea.

4.   Chicken breast fajitas (wholegrain tortilla) with red peppers and onions, green salad with half an avocado and peppermint or green tea.

5.   Lean grilled steak with steamed mixed vegetables and new potatoes. Peppermint or green tea.

6.   Brown rice pilaf with baked salmon, green salad and peppermint or green tea.

7.   Roast pork fillet, Mediterranean roasted vegetables, mashed potato (with skin) and peppermint or green tea.

8.   Chicken breast with onions and peppers in corn tortilla, mixed salad including half an avocado and peppermint or green tea.

9.   Wholegrain pasta with ratatouille (homemade is best onions, peppers, courgettes in tomato sauce) Sprinkle of parmesan cheese. Mixed Salad. Peppermint or green tea.

10. Cod (any white fish) in white sauce (made with semi-skimmed milk), new potatoes, carrots and two green vegetables. Peppermint or green tea

11. Roasted vegetable brochettes using onion, peppers, courgettes and aubergine. Brown rice mixed with a little fried onion (use a little olive oil in the pan). Broccoli. Peppermint or green tea.

12. Cottage Pie with minced chicken, onions, mushrooms and mashed potato with cabbage and carrots. Peppermint tea or green tea.

13. Roast Turkey, brown rice and onion, Roast Parsnips, courgettes and peas with gravy. Peppermint or green tea.

14. Whole grain spaghetti with tomato and basil sauce (homemade with pureed tomatoes, olive oil, onions and fresh basil). Peppermint or green tea.

14 Light Meal Options

These are intended for either lunchtime or evening depending on when you have your main meal.

Portion size is important and I use a large cereal bowl or soup bowl approximately 6 inches or 15 cm in diameter and 4 inches or 10 cm in depth. You will be having three snacks per day in addition so you will soon adjust to having slightly less at this mealtime.

Most of these can be prepared and stored in the fridge saving you time. Jacket potatoes can be wrapped in foil and rice and pasta salads keep well too. I do suggest that you prepare your salads at the time as fresh fruit and vegetables do lose much of their goodness when cut. The exception to this is the fresh fruit salad which is stored in unsweetened apple juice which can be stored for three or four days in an airtight container in the fridge.

1. Raw Vegetable salad with chopped jacket potato – drizzle of olive oil. Green tea.
2. Brown rice salad with onions, mushrooms, peas with half a chopped chicken breast, green tea.
3. Whole grain sandwich with chicken breast, drizzle of olive oil and seasoning, lettuce and tomato. Green or peppermint tea
4. Spanish omelette made with an egg, a little cold potato, chopped red peppers and onions. Can be made in the microwave without oil. Peppermint or green tea.
5. Homemade vegetable soup (can be made and frozen) Use onions, peppers, mushrooms, carrots and any green vegetable with a salt free vegetable stock cube. Season to taste and you can make spicy. One wholegrain or olive bread roll with olive oil. Green tea
6. Half an avocado with prawns in teaspoon of mayonnaise, green salad and piece of wholegrain bread. Green tea.
7. Raw vegetable salad with tin of tuna in brine. Corn tortilla. Green tea
8. Sugar Free baked beans on two slices of whole grain toast drizzled with olive oil. Green tea
9. Homemade gazpacho with pureed tomato, cucumber and onion. Small jacket potato with light cream cheese. Green tea
10. Corn tortilla wrap with lettuce, tomato and two rashers of lean bacon.
11. Small pizza base with 1 oz of grated cheddar, onion, tomato puree, asparagus tips and chopped chicken. Green tea.
12. Cold pasta salad (wholegrain) with chopped spring onions, broccoli, cucumber and tomato and fresh shrimp. Green tea.
13. Whole grain French bread with fresh baked salmon, cucumber and scrape of mayonnaise and seasoning. Green tea.
14. Two poached eggs and steamed asparagus on two slices of wholegrain toast.

Snacks

It is the turn of the snacks now and these are important as we often turn to high fat sugary options during the day for convenience. More than anything, substituting healthy alternatives into our diet can make a huge difference to both our weight and our well being.

It is important that you do not go more than two or three hours without eating something so that your body keeps working and using energy. You do not want your blood sugar dropping and by eating regularly throughout the day you will find that you are less tired and more inclined to do the exercise that you need.

I suggest making up your fresh fruit salad and putting it into a large sealed container in the fridge and make a habit of having one bowl with low fat yoghurt every day. This will give you at least two of your portions of fruit that you need. Make sure that you leave at least two hours after your main meal before eating the fruit salad as it digests very quickly and can cause acidity if it interferes with the digestion of tougher and more fibrous foods. I find that it is a very useful snack in the evening around an hour before I go to bed.

On that basis that takes care of one snack per day and here are some examples of others that you can take to work with you or in your handbag if you are out shopping etc. If you are out and do not have anything to hand then stop for a cup of tea and a piece of toast or toasted teacake.

- Eat mid-morning, mid-afternoon and about an hour before bedtime.
- One snack per day to be a cereal bowl of fresh fruit salad with low fat yoghurt.
- Have a cup of green, peppermint or black tea with the morning and afternoon snack.

I have given you sufficient examples for you to get the idea of what sort of snack we are looking at. Get creative and find foods that you enjoy and can fit into your lifestyle that are healthy and energy giving. Please avoid buying the so called healthy energy bars. They are usually laden with sugar and are not as healthy as they are made out to be.

You can however make your own cereal bars using oats, whole grain flour, dried fruits and honey so find a good recipe and adapt to keep healthy. These can be stored in an airtight container in your desk or at home and the only proviso is that you don't become so hooked that you cannot stop at one digestive sized cookie at a time!

17 Snack options

1. Bowl of fruit salad with low fat yoghurt every day.
2. Homemade cereal cookie with a cup of green tea.
3. Orange and apple
4. Banana and 6 walnut halves.
5. Half a melon with berries.
6. Two oatcakes with scrape of butter and marmite.
7. Two Ryvita with scrape of butter and jam.
8. Two large plums and 6 walnut halves.
9. Apple and Pear
10. Piece of wholegrain toast, drizzle of olive oil and sliced tomato.
11. Banana or other fruit smoothies with 400 ml of semi skimmed milk and teaspoon of honey.
12. Sunflower seeds unsalted (small handful)
13. Pumpkin seeds unsalted (small handful)
14. Pot of low fat live yoghurt.
15. Two Ryvita with light cream cheese and tomato.
16. Pot of low fat rice pudding. (You can make your own with cooked brown rice, semi Skimmed milk and honey)
17. Cold hard boiled egg and a banana.

Recipes to Help You Get Started

Healthy Meusli To Start the Day

The ingredients in this recipe will not only kick start your day but have been shown to boost your immune system, protect your heart and cardiovascular system, act as an anti-inflammatory and control your blood sugar levels. Include the Green Tea and the Orange Juice and you will be getting a good proportion of your nutritional needs for the day.

A Week's Supply
- 12 oz of oats
- 6 oz of sliced almonds
- 6 oz of chopped dried apricots
- 6 oz of chopped walnuts
- 4 chopped prunes
- 1 chopped fig
- 1 teaspoon of cinnamon

Serve with a fresh fruit of the day – peach, apple, banana, cherries, pears and a pot of natural yoghurt.

Brown Rice Pilaf

Our systems quickly store up toxins if we are not careful and this recipe is great for helping remove them from the body as well as give you a powerful nutritional punch. You can use every night as an accompaniment to your evening meal or as a light lunch option.
Four servings. You can freeze three portions and use as needed.

- 225 gm / 8 oz of brown rice (you can add some wild rice for flavour)
- 15 ml / 1 tbsp. olive oil.
- 750 ml / 1 ¼ pints of salt free vegetable stock.

- 1 large finely chopped onion.
- 10 chopped walnuts.
- 4 oz of finely chopped spinach or dandelion leaves.
- 1 crushed clove of garlic.
- Florets of broccoli washed and chopped.
- Salt and pepper to taste.

- Wash the rice under cold running water and drain.
- Heat your oil in a large pan and add the onion and the garlic and cook until soft and brown.
- Add the rice and stir in the stock.
- Bring to the boil, cover and simmer for 20-25 minutes.
- Stir in the chopped spinach or dandelion leaves, walnuts and seasoning.
- Serve with a garnish of raw broccoli.
- This is wonderful with a few ounces of turkey or salmon.

Stuffed Red Peppers With Walnuts

Here is a recipe that is packed with many of the nutrients needed to keep your circulatory system healthy and clear of blockages. Full of B-vitamins, vitamin C, fibre and essential fatty acids. If you wish you can add some lean meat, fish or chicken to the stuffing.

This is a recipe for 4 people or four portions if you want to freeze and use later.

- 4 large red peppers
- 1 large red onion
- 1 courgette chopped
- 4 oz of shitake mushrooms
- 4 oz of chopped walnuts
- 4 oz of finely chopped celery
- 2 oz of porridge oats.
- 2 large tomatoes finely chopped.
- 2 tablespoons of fresh chopped basil
- ½ teaspoon of pimiento
- 4 oz of grated Edam cheese.
- Salt and pepper to taste
- 2 tablespoon of olive oil.
- Optional extra. Add a chopped (cooked) chicken breast, lean lamb or fresh salmon.

The oven needs to be preheated to 180 C.

Put the oil, onion, celery, courgette and shitake mushrooms into a pan and cook for about 5 minutes gently. Stir in your tomatoes and cook for another 8 to 10 minutes stirring occasionally. Remove from the heat and stir in the oats, walnuts, basil and seasoning.

Cut the peppers in half lengthways and seed them. Either put into boiling water for two or three minutes or microwave in a steamer for the same time. Put them in a shallow ovenproof dish and fill each one with the vegetable mixture. Cover with foil and bake for 15 to 20 minutes and then remove foil. Put the grated Edam cheese over the top of each pepper and replace in the oven for another 5 to 10 minutes until the cheese has melted.

Serve with large spinach "super salad".

Banana, Orange and Walnut Salad

This recipe is a lovely accompaniment to fish, meat or chicken dishes and served with a spinach leaf salad. With the tomatoes, walnuts, bananas, oranges and spinach this is a great Superfood salad.

- 2 tablespoons of white wine vinegar
- Salt and white pepper to taste.
- 1 teaspoon of honey
- ½ a small onion very finely chopped.
- 2 tablespoons of olive oil.
- Juice of half a lemon
- 2 bananas peeled, sliced. (Sprinkle with the lemon juice)
- 2 large tomatoes quartered.
- 2 mandarin oranges peeled and segmented.
- 14 walnut halves

- Combine the vinegar, salt, pepper, honey and oil into a bowl.
- Toss the banana in the dressing.
- Add the tomatoes and the oranges and walnut halves.
- Arrange over a plate of young spinach salad leaves.

Turkey Fajitas for 6 People

I usually allow three tortillas per person and I also use the soft maize tortillas by Old El Paso as being the best and the largest for this dish.

There is nothing worse than a mean fajita. So I use plenty of lean turkey instead of beef or chicken or you can use large peeled prawns if you prefer.

Seasoning

I use this low salt recipe to sprinkle over the vegetables and meat during cooking.

- Paprika 5 teaspoons
- Chilli Powder 6 teaspoons
- Garlic Powder 2 teaspoons
- Ground Cumin 4 teaspoons
- Salt ¼ teaspoon
- Black pepper ¼ teaspoon.

Turkey Filling for Tortillas

- 2 whole turkey breasts, sliced into long strips.
- 2 large Red Peppers sliced lengthways into strips
- 2 large Green or yellow peppers sliced lengthways into strips
- 4 large Onions sliced into thick rings
- 18 soft corn or wheat tortillas.
- Olive Oil

In a large oven proof dish arrange all the vegetables in layers sprinkling a little of the seasoning onto each lager drizzle a little olive oil over the dish and put into a hot oven around 200 degrees for 10 minutes. Remove and add the strips of turkey so that they do not overlap and put the remaining seasoning over the entire dish. Drizzle with a little more olive oil and put back in the oven until the turkey is cooked thoroughly which is about 15 to 20 minutes.

Serve in the oven dish at the table.

Warm your tortillas, and a tip here is to put 6 each in a foil packet and pop in the oven for the last 5 minutes cooking time. Turn the oven off and leave two of the packets in there until you need them.

On the table you will need dishes of guacamole, salsa and Fromage Blanc. By all means use sour cream or Crème Fraiche is you are not worried about the calories. You can also serve grated cheese with the other dressings.

For anyone who has not eaten fajitas before, a teaspoon of each sauce is spread over a warm tortilla and then the peppers; onions and turkey mix is placed in the middle. The bottom end of the tortilla is folded towards the middle and the two sides are brought over to form a wrap. The whole thing is eaten with your hands.

I usually have a large bowl of the spinach salad on the table as well as it helps if the food is spicier for some people than normal.

You can substitute lean beef; chicken fresh peeled prawns in the recipe and adjust the cooking times slightly. If you are vegetarian then add your favourite vegetables and roasted these make a delicious alternative.

I had never eaten fajitas before I went to live in Texas twenty years ago. I use turkey or salmon, two of the superfoods regularly in the recipe and if you make your own guacamole and salsa with avocados, tomatoes and onions you will be using other superfoods in this great dish for entertaining or for a family meal.

Onion and Garlic Soups

I have chosen two soups which are ideal if you are suffering from a cold or the flu but are also an excellent way to use onions and garlic two or three times a week as a light lunch or supper. You can add cooked brown rice to the onion soup to make it more substantial but the creamy garlic soup is wonderful with whole grain, warm French bread.

These recipes are also great to include in any diet for the prevention of high cholesterol, blood pressure, raised blood sugar levels and inflammatory diseases such as arthritis or asthma.

Onion Soup

- 2 Tablespoons of olive oil.
- 2 lbs (1 kg) of peeled and thinly sliced onions
- 1 ½ pints (900 ml) of vegetable stock or water
- 2 garlic gloves, peeled and crushed
- Lemon juice
- Salt and black pepper to taste
- Chopped parsley or chives.

Heat the oil in a large saucepan, and then fry the onions until they are soft and deep golden brown but not burnt. Add the stock or water, garlic and a few drops of lemon juice. Bring the soup to the boil and let simmer for about 10 minutes. Season to taste with salt and pepper, sprinkle with the chopped parsley or chives and serve with warm wholegrain bread or add two tablespoons of cooked brown rice.

Creamy Garlic Soup

- 8 oz (225 gm) potatoes, scrubbed and diced but not peeled.
- 2 garlic bulbs broken into cloves.
- 1 tablespoon olive oil.
- Salt to taste
- 2 ½ pints (1.5 litres) water.

Put the potatoes and the garlic in a pan with the water, bring to the boil and allow to simmer for about 15 minutes or until the potato is tender. Allow to cool for 5 minutes and then liquidise and pour through a sieve into a clean pan. Add more water to adjust the consistency to your liking. Whisk in the olive oil and add salt to taste.

Gently reheat before serving with wholegrain bread or Pitta bread.

Entertaining

It is difficult not to dive into the crisp and the salted nut section of the supermarket when you are planning on entertaining guests. I have found it very useful to combine drink nibbles with the actual starter so that you get straight into the main meal or BBQ when you sit down.

Also if you invite people over for a drink only, it is lovely to be able to give them healthy and light snacks that can tide them over until they get home or go out to eat themselves.

If you have spent several hours in the kitchen preparing a wonderful meal for yourselves or if you are entertaining then you do not want to fill your guests up in advance so that they cannot do justice to your cooking.

I have some suggestions for some delicious alternatives to the usual salty and fatty products on the shelf.

Starting With Dips

Dips can be very fattening and filled with preservatives if you buy them ready prepared but I have a few that you can use either before dinner or as part of your main course. I also want to incorporate my superfoods and food pharmacy when possible and there is no better place to start than with Avocados and in particular Guacamole.

Avocados, as we talked about, are great for our cholesterol levels. Onions are anti-bacterial, anti-inflammatory, and have anti histamine properties as well as the levels of chromium that help stabilise insulin levels and help prevent blood platelets clumping leading to cardiovascular disease. The tomatoes are a perfect base or ingredient in any dips and they of course add their anti-oxidant properties as well as their protective lycopene that helps us fight cancer.

Guacamole

There are countless recipes for this Mexican sauce and when we lived in Texas every time we had a party several guests would arrive with their patented, world-winning version. Pre dinner or BBQ you can serve with raw vegetable crudities or with sliced warm Pitta bread. You can spice it up or down depending on your guest's and your own palates but do watch the chillies.

Recipe for 4 to 6 people.

- 2 large tomatoes, skinned, seeded and chopped.
- 2 tablespoons of finely chopped mild white onions or spring onions
- 2 large mashed avocado (leave until you have blended the rest of the ingredients)
- Salt to taste
- Juice of 1 large lemon
- 1 small red or green chilli depending on how spicy you would like it.
- Some fresh cilantro to taste.

Blend the onions, chillies, cilantro and salt in a processor, mix in the mashed avocado and the chopped tomatoes and put in a pretty bowl in the middle of your vegetables or Pitta bread. If you are going to use for your main course with fajitas then chill until you need.

Salsa as a Dip or to Accompany Fajitas

- 5 medium to large fresh tomatoes, skinned and chopped.
- 1 green pepper de-seeded and chopped very finely.
- 1 medium onion or two spring onions chopped finely.
- Juice of one lemon
- 1 small red or green chilli (optional)

- 1 clove of crushed garlic
- 1 tablespoon of fresh chopped cilantro leaves.
- Salt and pepper to taste.

Mix altogether and chill in the refrigerator.

The Appetisers

There are some classic tapas dishes that you can serve before dinner or BBQ that are light and easy to prepare and here are some of my favourites. Packed with anti-oxidants that make your dishes as colourful as possible.

Vegetable Brochettes

Depending on how many people you are serving you will need the following ingredients per brochette.

- Red pepper
- Aubergine,
- Courgette
- Button mushroom
- Cherry tomatoes
- Slice of onion.
- Olive oil, Pepper, Pimiento and salt

Cut all your vegetables into chunks except for the tomatoes. Thread them all through the wooden skewers. Lay on an ovenproof dish.

Mix your pepper, pimiento and salt together.

Drizzle your brochettes with olive oil and then sprinkle with your dry seasoning mix.

Your oven should be around the 175 to 200 mark and the brochettes will cook in around 15 minutes.

Stuffed Mushrooms

- Large washed mushrooms with the stalks removed and put to one side.
- 1 medium onion
- 1 small red pepper
- Small tinned tuna in brine or salmon drained and mashed.
- Fresh parsley finely chopped.

- 1 large tomato skinned and finely chopped.
- Olive oil.
- Salt and pepper to taste

Chop the stalks of the mushrooms and add to the other chopped ingredients and the seasoning. Blend in the tuna or salmon and refill the mushrooms. Drizzle with olive oil. Put in a preheated over at about 175 to 200 for about 10 minutes. Serve hot.

Aphrodisiacs?

I hope that having read through this book you are now convinced that you can definitely play a role in not only improving your sex life but more importantly deal with the underlying health issues that are most probably the cause of your dysfunction in the first place.

There is nothing new in history and certainly man (and woman) has tried since day one to maintain sexual attractiveness and performance. However aphrodisiacs achieved their reputations there is a definite link to nutrition as you will see in the this chapter.

Perhaps Adam thought the apple was an aphrodisiac when he offered it to Eve and certainly the belief that foods could stimulate and arouse us to passion has been honoured by both men and women since earliest recorded time.

It is a belief that is held across every race, culture and age group, which makes for interesting research into the subject.

Foods, herbs, spices and unfortunately certain animal parts have been considered to be stimulating over the ages and I am going to focus on food and herbs that are still readily available today in our supermarkets.

Aphrodisiacs were taken in the first instance to calm anxiety and therefore improve sexual performance. Having children was considered a necessity from both a moral and a religious perspective and so being at peak fertility was considered essential for both men and women.

Aphrodisiacs are broken down into two distinct functions. Nutritional to improve fertility and performance and stimulating to increase desire. Being poorly nourished will affect both semen and egg production and quality so it was considered important to eat nutritional packed foods such as seeds, roots and eggs, which were considered to contain sexual powers.

To stimulate desire it was thought that eating foods that resembled the sexual organs would produce the required result and of course there was always the hearsay element of mythology and fairy tales to establish credibility for one food or another. Many of the foods considered by the ancient civilisations such as Egypt, Greek and Roman to be aphrodisiacs are still available today, and we eat them on a regular basis. This makes it a little difficult to determine if the rocket, pistachio nuts, carrots and basil that you eat as part of your normal diet are acting as stimulants or not. At least most of us are no longer indulging in gladioli roots or skink lizard flesh although the French may well claim that their continued consumption of snails may have something to do with their reputation as the best lovers.

Before we take a look at some of the common foods that might be sexually stimulating we should just mention a few that might have an inhibiting effect on your libido.

Apparently eating too many lentils, lettuce, watercress, and water lilies might affect your performance although I suspect that there are more than a few rabbits that might disagree with that belief.

Some Foods That Are Considered to Be Aphrodisiacs

Aniseed was believed by the Egyptians, Greeks and the Romans to have very special properties and they sucked the seeds to increase desire. Aniseed was also favoured for its medicinal properties, which may explain its popularity as a sexual stimulant. It was used to reduce flatulence (not a particularly attractive condition) remove catarrh, acts as a diuretic and as an aid to digestion combined with other herbs such as ginger and cumin. One of its properties was to increase perspiration and one wonders if this additional heat was confused with an increase in desire. However if you are planning a romantic interlude avoid drinking it in tea form as it was considered a very effective insomnia cure.

Asparagus

Well regarded for its phallic shape and also for particular stimulating properties. It was suggested that you fed it to your lover over a period of three days either steamed or boiled. One explanation of its supposed success is that it acts as a liver and kidney cleanser and also a diuretic. After three days it is likely that you might feel more energetic and also have lost a couple of pounds, guaranteed to give anyone a boost sexual or otherwise.

Almonds

Long been considered the way to a girl's heart in particular their aroma, which is supposed to induce passion in a female. Almonds are incredibly nutritious, packed with vitamins, minerals, protein and healthy fat so there is no doubt that regular consumption of this and other nuts would be likely to improve overall general health and therefore fertility Almonds have been prepared in a number of ways over the ages but certainly the one that seems the most popular is marzipan, guaranteed to win over any sweet-toothed female, young or old.

Avocado

Historically, was regarded as an aphrodisiac mainly due to its shape. The Aztecs called the avocado tree "Ahuacuati" or testicle tree and when brought to Europe the Spanish called the fruit aquacate. Apart from the shape the fruit has a sensuous smooth texture and exotic flavour that stimulates all the senses. Again including avocados in your diet several times a week will contribute to your general health as well as possibly improving your love life.

The Banana

One of our healthy and medicinal foods. Obviously the shape played some part in its reputation as an aphrodisiac but it is very rich in potassium and B vitamins, which are both essential for healthy hormone production. Eating one banana is unlikely to enhance sexual performance but including them on a regular basis will certainly have you firing on all cylinders.

Cloves

Amongst other herbs and spices contain eugenol, which is very fragrant and aromatic. It has been used for centuries as a breath freshener, which may be hint to why in days before dental hygiene became so important eating it before a date was considered an aphrodisiac.

Chocolate

Like almonds, chocolate has long been regarded as an enticement to females and contrary to popular belief; Cadburys were not the inventors of this delicious if very addictive treat. The Aztecs called it the "nourishment of the Gods" probably because of the chemicals in chocolate that stimulate neurotransmitters in the brain that produce a feel good effect. It also stimulates the production of theobromine, which is related to caffeine and would no doubt stimulate performance in other areas.

Honey

Has been used medicinally for thousands of years and was considered essential as a cure for sterility and impotence. Even in medieval times less than scrupulous suitors would ply their dates with Mead, a fermented drink made from honey. This was also drunk by newly weds on their honeymoon probably acting to relax inhibitions and anxiety. Honey is wonderfully nutritious and again including it regularly in your diet is likely to improve your general state of health, which would lead to improved sexual performance.

Mace and Nutmeg

These contain myristicin and some compounds related to mescaline. Mescaline is found in Peyote cactus and has been used in South American and North American Indian cultures for over 2000 years as a hallucinogen. This might explain why the use of mace and nutmeg in aphrodisiac potions may have produced mild euphoria and loss of inhibitions. Hot milk and ground nutmeg has long been a night-time drink and now we know why.

Oysters

Well known for their aphrodisiac qualities in Roman times and their reputation continues today. There is some reference to their likeness to female sexual organs but the main thing going for oysters is their high content of Zinc. This mineral is essential for male potency but if you do not have a balanced diet with other sources of zinc, eating a dozen oysters from time to time is unlikely to give you the desired results.

Saffron

This has been used since the times of the ancient Greeks where it was harvested from the wild yellow crocus, flowers. Its use has since spread throughout the world and has been used for thousands of years as a medicine and as a perfume. It is said to be an excellent aid to digestion, increases poor appetite and being antispasmodic will relieve stomach aches and tension. More recently it has been used as a drug to treat flu-like infections, depression and as a sedative. As far as being an aphrodisiac is concerned its most important property is likely to be its ability to regulate menstruation which would of course help lead to a better chance of conception. It is generally a tonic and stimulant and being very versatile can be used in many dishes regularly in your diet.

There are many other foods, herbs and spices that have for one reason or another been associated with sexuality. These include liquorice, mustard, pine nuts, pineapple, strawberries, truffles, basil, garlic, ginger and vanilla. The one thing that is absolutely certain is that if you have an excellent balanced diet with plenty of variety you will be taking in all the above nutrients on a continuous basis and that will enable you to enjoy an active and full sex life. Adding a few of the above ingredients will certainly do you no harm and who knows you may be able to prove if they really are all they are cracked up to be.

Exercise and Flexibility

If you are already enjoying a moderate exercise regime then all that you perhaps might do with the following is review where you are now and how you might increase your fitness levels.

For anyone who lives a sedentary lifestyle then starting with the gentle breathing and flexibility exercises is a necessary place to begin. There is no point is stressing your body by attempting activities it is in no condition to take part in. It only leads to damage to your body and when you hurt you give up.

Spend as long as necessary on each stage of the fitness programme until you feel confident you can move onto the next. Each will be beneficial in its own way.

The Power of the Siesta

Sleep is as vital to humans as breathing, drinking water and following healthy diets. Before you contemplate your exercise programme to be healthy and sexy you need to ensure that you are also getting adequate rest.

We need the exercise and movement throughout the day to keep us supple and fit but you cannot run any operating system for 24 hours per day, 7 days per week for 70 or 80 years without carrying out essential maintenance.

If we are doing our bit we should be providing the body the raw materials it needs to process, manufacture and rebuild our bodies internally and externally. However, sleep is the missing ingredient that many of us are depriving our bodies of.

During the day our activities help our bodies to excrete toxins but the body also needs time to heal, rejuvenate and rest. Most of the day our body is focussing on keeping you upright and able to accomplish every task you set yourself including providing you with a functional immune system. At night your body can concentrate on cleansing and restoring all the operating functions ready for the next day.

For example the heart normally beats 82 times in a minute. That is 4,920 times an hour or 118,080 times a day. However when we are asleep our hearts beat around 60 beats per minute or lower. This means that for 8 hours of the day our heart will beat 28,800 instead of 39,360 times, which is a saving of 10,560 beats. If you multiply that over a year you will be saving nearly 4 million heartbeats. Take that onto our lifespan and your heart will have to work millions of heartbeats less, saving wear and tear on this vital organ.

The same principal applies to the rest of the body and its operating systems. Your lungs will work less as your breathing slows during the night. Your muscles will rest and recuperate and your brain will undergo diagnostic tests and repairs while you sleep.

Most mental disorders including depression and Alzheimer's are linked to various sleep disorders, some resulting from drugs used to control the disease or from changes in parts of the brain that normally regulate sleep patterns.

Going without sleep affects our mood and stress levels and this is the result of hormonal imbalances caused by lack of down-time for the body. The glands that produce these hormones such as the adrenal glands are on constant alert and have no chance to rest and rejuvenate. As in the case of a rowdy neighbour it is "one up, all up". The knock on effect of having all these hormones rampaging around the body is that nobody gets any rest leading to physical, mental and emotional problems.

Performance levels will decrease without proper sleep and our reactions and internal processes will be impaired. Research has shown that sleep deprivation has the same effect on driving performance as taking alcohol or drugs. People who do not get enough sleep become increasingly less sensitive to certain chemical reactions within the body and in the case of insulin this increases the risk to developing both diabetes and high blood pressure.

If you are constantly feeling tired then you will experience a corresponding reduction in your sex drive. Your sexual performance is reliant on not only a healthy diet but an efficient operating system. If your body is malnourished, tired and stressed it will concentrate on survival and the non-essential activities outside of simple survival will take a back seat.

If You Are Tired Then Your Body Is Trying To Tell You Something

Taking a nap is actually a way to catch up on your missing sleep. The most natural time for a nap is 8 hours after you have woken up in the morning and 8 hours before you go to bed. This way it is unlikely to affect your ability to fall asleep at night. Even 20 minutes can actually revitalise you and rest your body ready for another 8 hours of activity.

Make yourself comfortable, loosen your clothes and just close your eyes. Even if you do not fall asleep your body will relax and everything from your muscles to your brain will benefit.

Getting To Sleep at Night

Unless you are from a Mediterranean country and used to eating late each night from childhood, avoid having dinner just before you go to bed. At least leave an hour and if it has been very spicy then leave for at least two hours. I have no idea how anyone can go out for a night drinking, eat a curry and go to bed and not suffer a dreadful night's sleep.

Alcohol is a stimulant and whilst excessive amounts may make you sleepy it is going to wake you up four hours later with a raging thirst and a thumping headache. Once in while you may get away with it but if it is the norm you will become seriously sleep deprived.

Sitting up too late, watching an action thriller is not the best way to ensure a good night's sleep. Those of us who have dogs who need walking benefit from both the physical activity and the fresh air before hitting the pillow and if you can safely take a stroll at night then it is an excellent idea. In the following sections you will find some breathing and flexibility exercises. These are ideal for last thing at night as they will not only give you a boost of oxygen but will help relax your muscles and stretch your body before sleep.

Make sure that there is plenty of airflow in the bedroom and sleep in comfortable clothes. I have no idea how people manage in button up pyjamas as they must be so restrictive and you will be moving around quite a bit at night and getting tangled up in both bedclothes and your night clothes is going to disturb you.

I find that however late I go to bed, reading a few pages of a book is guaranteed to make me drop off. Many people have discovered their own sleep triggers over the years including warm baths with Epsom salts, herbal teas such as Kava Kava and

Valerian, and gentle music that drowns out the noise of neighbours or a snoring partner.

Earplugs are very useful particularly if you are sharing a bed with a snorer although you may miss the alarm clock in the morning.

If you are going to bed at more or less the same time every night you will find within a very short space of time that you will wake at about the same time every morning. In fact it is a good idea to follow the same sleep patterns all week rather than opt for a lie in at the weekend. It establishes a healthy downtime for the body and does not confuse it for two days every week.

Sleep is an essential part of a healthy lifestyle and increasingly research is showing that it is also vital for the development of our brains. Children who do not get sufficient sleep will develop behavioural and learning difficulties as well as compromise their immune systems and future health.

Keeping your children up with you late at night is not healthy as they need far more sleep than we do during their rapid growth spurts. Make sure that they have a nap during the day about half way through their active hours and get them into the habit of getting at least 10 hours sleep per night. When they are very young you will obviously be waking them for feeds and then for potty training but you must always try and ensure that they are kept calm and are put back down as quickly as possible. This will also be healthier for you as this is the time when most parents are likely to suffer from sleep deprivation. The next crisis for those of you with teenagers is when they fail to return before 2.00 in the morning.

Stages of Sleep

There are a number of different stages of sleep and it is important that you go through the entire cycle to reap all the benefits.

There are two main phases. In phase one you will be going through Non-Rapid Eye Movement Sleep or NREM. There are different stages within this phase which naturally lead you to phase two or Rapid Eye Movement sleep or REM.

PHASE ONE – NREM

Stage One. This is the lightest stage of sleep and although your main senses are turned down they are not off completely and you can be disturbed by certain noises such as snoring, dogs barking or doors slamming.

Stage Two. If you get into this stage you will fall deeper asleep and your heart rate and temperature will begin to level out and drop. This stage represents about half your night's sleep.

Stage Three and Four are the deepest stages of NREM and represent about 15% of your nights sleep. Your breathing will slow; your temperature will drop further as will your blood pressure.

PHASE TWO – REM

After about 30 minutes in stage four NREM sleep you begin to move back to stage one and two where your brain will become more active and you will begin to dream. If you are woken up at this point in the cycle you are likely to remember the dream you were experiencing at the time. If you have reached one of the NREM stages then you are not as likely to recall anything when you wake up.

This cycle of phase one and two takes approximately 90 minutes and then begins again. To really benefit from this combination of rest and activity you need to complete at least 5 cycles during the night. This adds up to approximately 8 hours of sleep. If you only manage one or two cycles then your brain and body will not have completed its cleansing process and you will feel tired. If this becomes the norm you will begin to notice the symptoms of sleep deprivation.

Sleep is as essential as air, water and food and if you are not currently enjoying a good night's sleep then you need to work towards finding a solution.

Deep Breathing Exercises

BREATHING

Breathing correctly and taking in the right amount of Oxygen for our body can help you relax and reduce stress. It will improve your skin tone, reduce stress and improve your sex life. You will sleep better and in some cases lose weight.

More importantly many functions of the body, including the essential elimination of waste and toxins is dependent on our breathing. 70% of our elimination is through breathing, yet most people only use 20% of their lung capacity. This causes a build up of toxins which lead to disease and chronic illnesses associated with old age. Most bacteria and viruses do not thrive in an oxygen rich environment.

Our lungs are a tool that we can learn to use effectively at no cost and without taking in suppressive drugs that can cause us long term damage.

A few minutes each day spent in a deep breathing exercise and learning to breathe correctly using the lungs full capacity will have lasting benefits.

As far as losing weight is concerned achieving an aerobic state means getting enough Oxygen into the bloodstream to convert fuel to burn fat. This does not necessarily mean racing around breathing as hard as you can manage. What it does mean is achieving optimum breathing in gentle but effective exercises.

Breathing correctly can also release endorphins into the brain. Anything from panic attacks to migraine headaches can be improved by increasing Oxygen into the system.

It may take some practice but after a few days you will be amazed at the sort of power you can achieve working with your body's own capabilities.

My thanks to James Jewell, Yoga Master, for the following breathing exercises.

Some of the Benefits To the Whole Body by Breathing Correctly

We take breathing so much for granted that it may surprise you to know how many of our bodily functions are reliant on this automatic process.

THE RESPIRATORY SYSTEM
- Gives you more energy.
- Reduces mental and physical fatigue.
- Reduces chest pains caused by tight muscles, the tension causing anxiety of "heart attack potential" is reduced.
- Aids in relief of many long-term respiratory difficulties such as asthma and bronchitis.
- Reduces need for artificial stimulants and many harmful prescription drugs.
- Helps eliminate waste from the body

CIRCULATORY SYSTEM
- Improves blood circulation and relieves congestion.
- Increases supply of oxygen and nutrients to cells throughout the body. Major organs such as brain and eyes need plenty of oxygen.

- Eases the strain on the heart by increasing oxygen to the heart.
- Helps increase the supply of blood and nutrients to muscle blood and bones.

The Nervous System
- Better breathing can calm or stimulate the nervous system, balance or unbalance brain hemispheres, depending on the technique.

The Digestive System
- Diaphragmatic action acts as a pump to massage the internal organs, aiding their function.

Endocrine System
- Helps push the movement of lymph throughout the body, which helps eliminate toxic wastes and strengthen the immune system

The Urinary System
- Shallow breathing puts stress on other organs of elimination.
- Better breathing can reduce oedema, (swelling of the body) by eliminating fluids thorough the breath.

The Skin
- CO_2 waste is eliminated more directly through breath.
- Wrinkles can be lessened due to improved circulation and blood oxygen flow.
- Radiant skin is a sign of good oxygenation

Movement
- Relaxes muscle spasm and relieves tension.
- Releases and reduces muscular tension that eventually may cause structural problems.
- Helps increase flexibility and strength of joints; when you breathe easier you move easier.
- Facilitates stretching of connective tissue, which prevents formation of adhesions and reduces the danger of fibrosis.
- Can partially compensate for lack of exercise and inactivity due to habit, illness or injury.

Breathing Exercise To Relax and Cleanse The Body – Five Minutes a Day If Possible

There are 4 parts to every breath.
1. The inhale
2. A moments pause
3. The exhale
4. And another natural moment's pause before the next inhale.

The exhale usually longer than the inhale.

Morning Breathing Exercise

- Stand with your arms relaxed by your side, with the whole body relaxed and still. Your posture should be straight but not held taut. The shoulders rolled back and down to open the chest and release neck/shoulder tension.
- As you inhale slowly lift the arms out and up above your head with palms parallel.
- As you exhale release the arms back down gently to your sides. So not only do you receive a gentle stretch to wake you up, but also there is more space in the body to take a deeper inhalation. It is very simple but very effective.
- The most important thing is to unite the length of the inhale with the rise of the arms so that when the arms reach the furthest point above the head we have completed the inhale; there is a tiny pause, then the exhale down, slowly lowering the arms.
- When they reach your side the exhale is finished. Generally the exhale is longer than the inhale as you are ridding the body of impurities with it.
- Then a little pause. The movements follow the breath, like surfing a wave. Don't rush the moves or you will get tense, better to do them slow and relaxed with total concentration, better still outside (on a beach) or in front of an open window to receive all that fresh air!
- Practice for several minutes or at least 12 times. Better to do 12 mindful breaths then 25 rushed ones. Quality versus quantity.
- If you suffer with high blood pressure and or restrictive shoulder/arm movements, better to take the arms up only as far as the shoulder height.

EVENING BREATHING EXERCISE

The purpose here is to encourage slow, deep breathing using as much of the lungs as possible.

- Lie down on your back on the floor. If you have lower back pain, better to have your knees resting up over on sofa or chair. If your head doesn't relax onto the ground easily, use a cushion.
- Start with your hands on your lower belly, fingers pointing down to groin. Notice how you are breathing. The breath reflects our mental, physical and emotional state.
- After several minutes consciously encourage the beginning of the breath into the belly to feel the hands rise with the inhale and relax down with the exhale. So you are using the abdomen to breathe. Normally this should happen spontaneously, but all too often with stress many people breath only using the upper chest.
- Do this for several minutes, then place the arms out in a cross, shoulder height with palms up. Now there is more room to take the breath up into the middle lungs, feeling the movement of the ribcage move, outwards and upwards. But you still begin each breath down deep in the belly. Do this for several minutes, relaxing the body on the exhale.
- Last of all; slide your arms higher up above your head which is relaxing on the floor. If you can't do this due to tension or injury, leave them where they were in a cross. The purpose of this move is to now bring more space and awareness to the upper chest towards the base of the throat. There is little movement here compared to the ribs, but you should feel the rising of the chest and clavicle bones to the throat and chin at the peak of the inhale, just before we exhale.
- So you now have 3 places to breathe into, the abdomen, the ribs and the upper chest to make one long, deep, satisfying breath. Feel each of the 3 places as the breath flows up the trunk as one long wave. As you exhale the wave retreats back down to the lower abdomen. Remember to feel the slight pause between inhales and exhales, but don't hold the breath.
- Try and practise this for at least 5 minutes, but 10 is better. It also helps improve your posture with the back flat and the arms out.

Gentle Exercise

As you will have seen in the previous section on correct breathing, you do not have to race around doing aerobics and playing squash to obtain the aerobic (oxygen) benefits you need.

If you are doing the breathing exercises and combining them with a walking programme that increases in intensity over a period of weeks you will be getting all the benefits you need.

For example it can reduce the risk of Coronary heart disease, strokes, diabetes, High Blood Pressure, Bowel Cancer, Alzheimer's disease, Osteoporosis, Arthritis and stress. All these conditions are ones we have talked about as the leading causes of ageing so walking is definitely up there as an exercise of choice. Obviously it is key if you are trying to lose weight and if you are particularly overweight, walking is the safest and most sensible way to exercise to begin with.

Apart from increasing bone and muscular strength it will also increase your joints range and flexibility. One of the drawbacks to middle age sex is that we are certainly not as flexible as we were in our 20's and 30's. There is nothing worse than contemplating leisurely lovemaking when your knees and hips are painful and you are out of breath after five minutes. Following the breathing exercises above will certainly improve your stamina and after a few weeks of incorporating the following flexibility exercises you will be pleasantly surprised at how youthful you feel.

Flexibility

We can maintain our flexibility and actually improve it as we get older. The main reason we get stiff as we age is because we stop moving our bodies into different positions. The body is designed to move, not to stay sitting or slouching the majority of the time! As with everything, if we don't use, it we lose it! The more flexibility and space we have in our bodies, the deeper the breaths can be and the better our ability to get rid of harmful toxins.

Here are three simple exercises to incorporate with your breathing exercises to increase flexibility and joint health.

3 simple postures

No 1. STANDING EXTENDED, MOUNTAIN POSE

- In a standing position as in the breathing exercise, you raise your arms on inhale, but also lift your heels to stretch the whole body upwards, whilst on tip toe. On the exhale you lower your arms slowly and your heels back to the floor. It is also a balance so it helps develops concentration and focus. Keep your eyes fixed on a point during the exercise. Repeat 7/8 times.

No 2. CAT POSE GOOD FOR ALL ROUND SPINAL FLEXIBILITY

- Come onto all fours. Hands under the shoulders, knees under the hips. Imagine what a cat looks like when it gets up to stretch after napping. It arches its back up into the air.
- So now with the back flat, exhale and arch the spine up, dropping your head relaxed. The whole abdomen is drawn up to support the spine up. Pause to feel the stretch. Inhale slowly flatten the back again. Pause. Exhale; slowly arch the spine up again etc. Always working slowly, enjoying the move. At least 8 times.
- No 3. Knees to chest. Good for relaxing and toning lower back and belly.
- This posture is universally recognised as one of the best to help lower back pain.
- Lying down. Inhale your arms back above head; exhale with your right knee to chest with hands around it, to draw it in closer. Inhale arms back, leg back on ground. Exhale left knee up with hands on it and continue as this 8 times to each knee. Then 8 more times with both knees coming to chest together.
- Then relax still for at least several minutes to appreciate what you have done and enjoy the benefits of the movements and deep breathing.

A Six Week Walking Programme

After following the healthy eating programme and following the breathing and flexibility exercises for two or three weeks it is time to embark on a more active exercise programme.

If you have any kind of physical problem with your legs, ankles, knees or hips then make sure that you take this next stage slowly and carefully. If you have a serious problem then you should stay on the breathing and flexibility exercises but include a midday session as well.

If you are fit enough to begin a walking programme then make sure you have comfortable shoes that support both your feet and ankles.

You should start with a 20-minute walk at least five times a week. Brisk walking is the best and you need to be slightly breathless, as this is the point at which you will be fat burning and helping your body to lose fat and form muscle.

If you are currently walking for 20 minutes per day then you need to measure the distance you are walking. Over the next 6 weeks raise the time you walk to 40 minutes per day and you can split that if you like.

Walking uphill during part of your walk will increase your intensity but the right walking speed for you depends on your age and sex. To give you an idea of overall fitness levels I will give you some speeds that you should be aiming for.

Speed and Distance
- Under age 40 you would be FIT if you were walking between 2.75 miles and 3.25 miles in 40 minutes.
- If you are between 40–55 years old you would be FIT if you were walking between 2.75 and 3 miles in 40 minutes.
- If you are between 55-75 years old you would be FIT if you walked between 2.5 and 2.75 miles in 40 minutes.

Measure your walking distances. Drive the car along the route or buy a pedometer – and then try to decrease the time it takes you to walk that particular route over a period of weeks.

Do not overdo it – this is not a challenge but a gradual way to increase your level of fitness and health over a period of weeks not days.

JOGGING
Walking as an easy and safe start to getting your essential exercise. You should spend several weeks getting to the fittest level for walking before attempting to jog and several weeks again before you start running.

Like walking, jogging will improve muscle tone including the heart muscle, it will build strength and flexibility although you may not believe that in the first few weeks and it will relieve stress. Your risk to muscles and joints is higher with jogging and you will have to spend more on proper running shoes and spend longer preparing for this level of exercise.

Jogging is still a relatively gentle exercise but it is more aerobic than walking and will burn off more calories than brisk walking. To give you a rough idea of how many you will burn off a person weighing 160 lb (73 kilos) walking briskly at 4 mph (6.4 kph) would burn 375 calories per hour. If they were to jog at just 5 mph (8 kph) they would burn 750 calories per hour.

PREPARATION

It is extremely important to make sure that your muscles are warmed up before attempting to jog. To be honest if you are more than two stone overweight and have not jogged before you should continue walking and increase both the speed at which you walk and the distance until you reach a weight that is suitable.

Jogging puts strain on the back, hips, knees and ankles and if you are overweight just carrying the excess pounds is more than enough stress for your joints without adding the additional pressure of jogging or running.

As with walking it is best to start aerobically, which means that you will be just out of breath and not gasping for air. The rule of thumb is that you should be able to hold a conversation while you exercise and this way you can be sure you are burning fat.

Warm up with a fast walk and some light stretching paying particular attention to your calf muscles, which will be taking most of the strain.

Keep your back straight and your shoulders back. Push off from your toes and land on the ball of your foot. Let your arms swing naturally at your side.

It is better to walk and jog alternately over your usual walking route so that you have a reasonable time target. If the distance is two miles and you normally cover this in 30 minutes aim to walk 100 steps and jog 100 steps and aim to finish in 26 minutes. This will equate to 4½ mph (7.2 kph) and increase of ½ mile per hour. Train at least three times a week and aim to be walking/jogging the same distance in 2 minutes less each week.

Gradually change the pacing so that you are walking 100 steps and jogging 120, 140, 160 etc. until you are jogging the entire distance comfortably and in no pain.

Make sure that you stretch all your muscles including those in your upper body when you finish.

Equipment

Invest in a pair of shoes that are suitable for jogging. I suggest getting professional advice on style and fitting from an athletic shop and also buy some athletic socks from them as these will help to prevent blistering. Rubbing Vaseline into your feet before putting your socks on is also helpful in preventing blisters and soaking your feet in warm salty water and drying them carefully after jogging will also prevent bacterial infections.

Always carry a bottle of water with you and do not run in the heat of the day. Stay hydrated as you will be losing not just sweat but essential salts and nutrients that will sap your energy. You may find on longer jogs that you need a cereal bar along the route and it is always a good idea to have eaten some carbohydrate a couple of hours before the run.

After the run you will find a banana and water a very good way to put some energy and fluids in fast.

Jog Safely

If you cannot jog in a designated pedestrian area always face oncoming traffic. Wear a reflective strip and light coloured clothing particularly in poor light. Do not jog alone in isolated areas for safety reasons and also in case you suffer an injury.

Vary your route and always try to jog with a friend. If you are alone carry a bum bag with plasters, a whistle, your keys, some form of identification and a mobile phone.

Once you have been jogging for several weeks and complete a satisfactory distance in a reasonable time you might like to move your exercise up a notch and begin running which will take you from 5–6 mph (8–11 kph) to 8–10 mph (13–16 kph) and entering some amateur competitions.

Afterword

After reading this lengthy health manual, you still of course have a choice. You can embark on a programme that will improve your health, stamina and ultimately, perhaps, your lifespan. Or you can still go ahead and take the little blue pill.

All that I ask is that you make sure you do go and have a full medical examination first with your doctor. Even young men may have underlying heart defects that might cause a problem if combined with the ingredients in any of the sexual enhancers.

There are a number of medical reasons why your doctor would prescribe medication to treat erectile dysfunction. Any other use has to be described as recreational and, like any other recreational drug, there are side effects. Some could be fatal.

Do not become a statistic.

As I have said many times, your body is your greatest asset and if you do not treat it with respect it cannot support you for a long and active lifetime.

Also by Sally Georgina Cronin

Just an Odd Job Girl
ISBN 978-1-9055997-12-3

Size Matters
ISBN 978-1-9055997-02-4

Just Food for Health
ISBN – 978-1-905597-23-9

Media Training – The manual
ISBN 978-1-905597-31-4

Sam, A Shaggy Dog Story
ISBN 978-1-905597-35-2

Just an Odd Job Girl

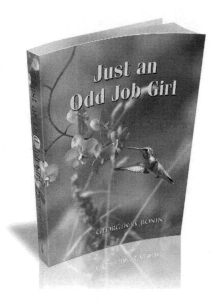

ISBN 978-1-905597-12-3
www.moyhill.com £6.99

Imogen was fifty!

She had been married to Peter for over twenty years and having brought up her children she was living in a wonderful house, with money and time to spare.

Suddenly, she finds herself "traded-in" for a younger model, a 'Fast-Tracker'. Completely devastated, she retreats to a small house on the edge of Epping Forest, where she indulges in binge eating and self-deprecation. Finally, when she can no longer fit into her clothes, and there seems to be no hope, she discovers a way forward.

Helped by a new friend, she rediscovers herself, making a journey to her past that enables her to move on to her future.

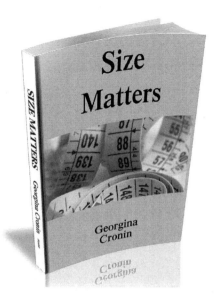

ISBN 978-1-9055997-02-4
www.moyhill.com £12.95

I wanted to find answers to explain how I had managed to eat and starve myself to 330 lbs This book is my story, but it is also the blueprint of the program that you will be following.

If any of these feels familiar
this book is definitely for you

- You can't take a bath because you can't get out again
- You don't even fit sideways into the shower
- You get desperate late at night when the chocolate shops are shut
- You are ashamed to take your clothes off in front of yourself
- You don't fit into airline seats and have to have a seat belt extension
- You struggle to get out of the car
- You can barely walk 10 minutes down the road
- You can't fit into public toilets
- People ask you when the baby is due
- You hate shop assistants coming into the too-small changing rooms
- You have stopped doing everything you once loved to do
- You have stopped sharing activities with the ones you love
- You are obsessed with where your next food is coming from
- You crave sweet foods
- You wish it would all go away

Just Food For Health

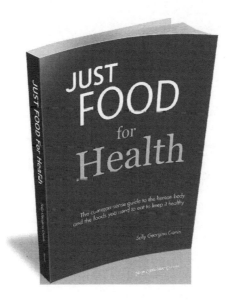

ISBN – 978-1-905597-23-9
www.moyhill.com £15.95

A new guide to a healthy lifestyle
by Sally Georgina Cronin.

'Just food for Health' is a comprehensive and common-sense guide to the body and the foods we need to eat to keep it healthy. Intended for the whole family, it covers not only how the body and major organs such as the heart and lungs, liver and kidneys function but what foods are necessary to keep them healthy at all ages.

The modern diet is filled with processed foods, high in sugars and unnatural fats. It is no wonder that, despite amazing advances in medical science, we still have far too many diseases that are lifestyle related.

The book also covers seasonal illnesses, dangers in our food such as additives, how to detox safely and healing foods and herbs.

Whether you want to lose weight safely and permanently or would like to make healthy changes to your diet and lifestyle, *'Just food for Health'* informs you how.

Media Training: The Manual

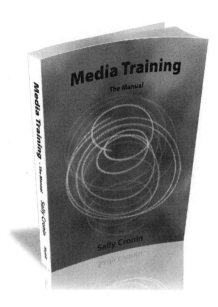

ISBN 978-1-905597-31-4
Print version £4.95 e-Book £ 2.99

A quick reference manual for anyone who needs the deliver their message via "the Media", TV, Radio, Print.

It is rumoured that the art of communication has been lost but actually it has simply been adapted and expanded to suit the new technologies. However, we still use our voices and radio and television are very powerful tools that can enable us to reach hundreds or even thousands of people in the space of a few minutes.

Those few minutes can have an enormous impact. By reaching out and engaging with an audience you can increase sales, sell your latest book, raise more funds for your charity or inform the public about an event or important community issue.

This guide to media training is about opening the door to that opportunity and making the most of the experience.

Sam, A Shaggy Dog Story

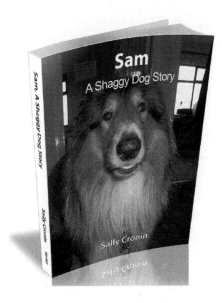

ISBN 978-1-905597-35-2
£7.49 Print
£3.59 e-Book

The Story of Sam and his friends

Millions of families around the World believe that their pet, dog or cat is most intelligent, beautiful and loyal friend that anyone could have. And they are absolutely right.

From the first moment that I met Sam, when he was just three weeks old, his personality and charm shone from his button eyes. Like many pet owners, we were convinced he understood every word we spoke and he actually could say one or two himself. Rather than tell his story from our perspective I have given him a voice and let him tell his own.

I can only imagine what he really thought about his two and four-legged friends but I do hope he loved us as much as we adored him and the time he spent with us shining brightly in our lives.

If only our pets could talk how much richer the world would be and funnier.